MIND THE GAPS

CASES IN GYNAECOLOGY, SEXUAL AND REPRODUCTIVE HEALTH

T0195334

MIND THE GAPS

CASES IN GYNAECOLOGY, SEXUAL AND REPRODUCTIVE HEALTH

Edited by

Shreelata Datta, MD, MRCOG LLM, MBBS, BSc (Hons)
Consultant Obstetrician and Gynaecologist, London
King's College London
UK

Usha Kumar, MBBS, MD, FRCOG, FFSRH
Consultant in Sexual and Reproductive Health, King's College
Hospital NHS Foundation Trust, London
UK

ELSEVIER

Elsevier
1600, John F. Kennedy Blvd.
Ste 1800
Philadelphia, PA 19103- 2899

MIND THE GAPS: CASES IN GYNAECOLOGY,   ISBN: 978-0-7020-8250-4
SEXUAL AND REPRODUCTIVE HEALTH

Notice

Practitioners and researchers must always rely on their own experience
and knowledge in evaluating and using any information, methods,
compounds or experiments described herein. Because of rapid advances
in the medical sciences, in particular, independent verification of
diagnoses and drug dosages should be made. To the fullest extent of the
law, no responsibility is assumed by Elsevier, authors, editors or
contributors for any injury and/or damage to persons or property as a
matter of products liability, negligence or otherwise, or from any use or
operation of any methods, products, instructions, or ideas contained in
the material herein.

Printed in Poland

Last digit is the print number: 9 8 7 6 5 4 3 2 1

Content Strategist: Alexandra Mortimer
Content Development Specialist: Veronika Watkins
Senior Project Manager: Manchu Mohan
Design: Ryan Cook
Graphics Coordinator: Narayanan Ramakrishnan
Marketing Manager: Deborah Watkins

Contents

List of Contributors

Nuala Coyle BA (hons) BMBS (hons)
Trainee in Obstetrics & Gynaecology
King's College Hospital
London, UK

Shruti Batham MBBS, MD, MRCOG, MFSRH
Specialty Doctor,
Kings College Hospital NHS Foundation Trust, London, UK

Shreelata Datta MD, MRCOG LLM, MBBS, BSc (Hons)
Consultant Obstetrician and Gynaecologist, London
King's College London
UK

Sai Gnanasambanthan MBBS, BSc (Hons), MRCOG, AICSM
Obstetrics & Gynaecology South London Trainee Registrar (ST5)
Lewisham & Greenwich NHS Trust, University Hospital Lewisham,
London, UK

Anna Graham MBBS, BA (Hons), MFSRH
Specialty Registrar in Community Sexual and Reproductive
Health, King's College Hospital NHS Foundation Trust,
London, UK

Usha Kumar MBBS, MD, FRCOG, FFSRH
Consultant in Sexual and Reproductive Health, King's College
Hospital NHS Foundation Trust, London, UK

Rupa Kumar BA (Hons) MB BChir (Cantab), Foundation Year 2
Doctor, Surrey and Sussex Healthcare NHS Trust, Redhill, UK

Rudiger Pittrof MSc, MRCOG, MFSRH, DipGUM, DTM&H, FHEA
Consultant in Community Sexual Health and HIV, Guy's
and St Thomas' NHS Foundation Trust, London, UK

Annette Thwaites MEng MA (Cantab) MSc MB BChir
Academic Clinical Fellow in Sexual and Reproductive Health
(SRH), Institute for Women's Health, University College London
Specialty Registrar in Community Sexual and Reproductive
Health, King's College Hospital NHS Foundation Trust, London, UK

Nektaria Varouxaki MRCOG, Diploma in Fetal Medicine
Senior Registrar in Obstetrics and Gynaecology
King's College Hospital NHS Trust, PRUH site, London, UK

Acknowledgements

We would like to thank our colleagues who have helped make this book what it is. It's been great working with you all, and your input has been invaluable.

A huge thank you to the team at Elsevier who have provided us with constant support to meet looming deadlines and worked with us with extreme patience during a very unique pandemic era.

Finally, we are extremely grateful to our friends and families for their unwavering encouragement and faith in us throughout the preparation of this book.

Preface

Modern medicine involves strict training programmes for health professionals. However, when working in the clinical environment, patients often present with clinical and ethical dilemmas that we may not always have come across in our training or in our practice. This book aims to address some common problems that we see regularly in gynaecology, sexual and reproductive health. It is designed to provide direction on subjects that are peripheral to a specialty but have a significant impact on patients' lives nonetheless and require our expertise and intervention. With the book written by doctors specialising in obstetrics, gynaecology and sexual health, we hope it will be a helpful resource to hospital doctors, general practitioners, nurses, allied healthcare professionals and students alike. We welcome feedback from readers so that we can make sure the next edition of this book is even more useful.

Dr. Shreelata Datta and Dr. Usha Kumar provided editorial oversight for Chapters 1–16 and 17–26 respectively.

List of Abbreviations

AED	antiepileptic drug
ART	antiretroviral therapy
ARV	antiretroviral
BMD	bone mineral density
BMI	body mass index
BPAD	bipolar affective disorder
cGIN	cervical glandular intraepithelial neoplasia
CHC	combined hormonal contraception
CIN	cervical intraepithelial neoplasia
COCP	combined oral contraceptive pill
CSF	cerebrospinal fluid
Cu-IUD	copper intrauterine device
DMPA	depo-medroxyprogesterone acetate
DNA	deoxyribonucleic acid
EC	emergency contraception
EE	ethinylestradiol
EHC	emergency hormonal contraception
EIAED	enzyme-inducing antiepileptic drug
FBC	full blood count
FGM	female genital mutilation
FIGO	International Federation of Gynecology and Obstetrics
FSH	follicle stimulating hormone
FVS	foetal varicella syndrome
GIC	gender identity clinic
GMC	General Medical Council
GnRH	gonadotrophin-releasing hormone
GP	general practitioner
GAS	gender-affirming (reassignment) surgery
HAART	highly active antiretroviral therapy
HCP	healthcare professionals
HFI	hormone free interval
HIV	human immunodeficiency virus
HPV	human papilloma virus
HRT	hormone replacement therapy
HSUPT	highly sensitive urine pregnancy test
HSV	herpes simplex virus
Ig	immunoglobulin
IMP	progestogen-only implant
IRIS	immune reconstitution inflammatory syndrome
IUC	intrauterine contraception
IUD	intrauterine device
IUS	intrauterine system
LAM	lactational amenorrhoea method
LARC	long-acting reversible contraception

LGV	lymphogranuloma venereum
LH	luteinising hormone
LMP	last menstrual period
LNG-IUS	levonorgestrel-releasing intrauterine system
MH	mental health
MRSA	methicillin-resistant *Staphylococcus aureus*
OSFED	other specified feeding or eating disorder
PCOS	polycystic ovary syndrome
PCR	polymerase chain reaction
PEPSE	postexposure prophylaxis after sexual exposure
PI	protease inhibitor
PID	pelvic inflammatory disease
PMB	postmenopausal bleeding
PMS	premenstrual syndrome
POP	progestogen only pill
QS	quick start
RVVC	recurrent vulvovaginal candidiasis
SARC	short acting reversible contraception
SDI	subdermal implant
SHBG	sex hormone binding globulin
SPC	Summary of Product Characteristics
SRH	sexual and reproductive health
SSRI	selective serotonin reuptake inhibitor
STI	sexually transmitted infection
STOP	surgical termination of pregnancy
TOC	test of cure
TSS	toxic shock syndrome
TVUSS	transvaginal ultrasound scan
UPSI	unprotected sexual intercourse
VTE	venous thromboembolism
VZIG	varicella zoster immunoglobulin

Recurrent Thrush

SAI GNANASAMBANTHAN • SHREELATA DATTA

Case

A 56-year-old woman with a body mass index (BMI) of 33 kg/m^2 presented with her fifth episode of what appeared to be thrush over a period of 8 months. She complained of dyspareunia as well as a white, thick discharge. She also complained of urinary frequency. Urine dipstick showed glucose 2+. Swabs were taken and she was commenced on oral fluconazole 150 mg every third day for 14 days. The swabs confirmed the diagnosis of heavy growth of *Candida albicans*. Once her initial treatment was completed, maintenance treatment was started for 6 months. Investigations for diabetes confirmed a diagnosis of noninsulin-dependent diabetes mellitus, and the patient was referred to a dietician for dietary glucose control and weight loss. At her 6 months' review, the patient had no further episodes and her blood glucose was under control.

Introduction and epidemiology

Recurrent thrush or recurrent vulvovaginal candidiasis (RVVC) is inflammation of the vulva or vagina or both, caused by superficial fungal infection, usually *Candida albicans*. However, roughly 10% to 20% of other Candida species can be identified as the causing pathogen. It is termed "recurrent" when a patient presents with four or more episodes in 1 year with at least partial resolution of symptoms between occurrences. Roughly 5% of women who present with a single episode will develop recurrent disease.[1] Predisposing factors include being immunocompromised or having uncontrolled diabetes mellitus, or any disturbance to the vaginal flora (with certain antibiotics). With maintenance treatment, around 90% of women will remain disease free at 6 months and 40% at 1 year. Thrush presents in men and women and can occur in the genital area as well as armpits, groin and between fingers.

Clinical presentation: signs and symptoms

Although the infection is harmless, it can be uncomfortable. Patients usually complain of itching or irritation around the vagina, with soreness or stinging during sexual intercourse or urination. On examination, there may be a white discharge (like cottage cheese) visible, which does not usually smell. However this is not always present, and it may just be an erythematous, painful rash that is visible, which may not be visible on darker skin.

Investigations

Women suspected to have the condition should have vaginal swabs taken to confirm thrush and rule out unusual pathogens. Microscopy, culture and sensitivity should be performed on the specimen. Measuring vaginal pH, if resources are available, can differentiate between Candida (pH $\leq$4.5), bacterial vaginosis (pH >4.5), or Trichomonas vaginalis (pH >4.5). Reversible causes of RVVC, such as diabetes mellitus, antibiotic use and other immunosuppressive disorders and medication, need to be identified. However, in most women, no predisposing cause can be found.[1,2]

Management

Treatment of the condition aims to control rather than cure the infection. Simple conservative measures include advice on avoiding bubble baths or spermicides that alter vaginal flora, avoiding nylon underwear or tight-fitting clothing, having antifungal treatment prescribed when taking antibiotics if this is identified as a predisposing factor, and advising lubrication use during intercourse, as friction could again cause minor damage to the vaginal wall, allowing the Candida species to thrive.

Although short courses of oral or topical azole therapy do work well for each episode, a longer induction course of 10 to 14 days of intravaginal or oral fluconazole 150 mg, every third day (giving a total of three doses), may work better at keeping symptoms controlled. Following this initial treatment, oral fluconazole 150 mg weekly or intravaginal clotrimazole 500 mg weekly for 6 months is usually the first-line therapy for maintenance, or a prescription for 'treatment as required' of either fluconazole 150 mg weekly or intravaginal clotrimazole 500 mg weekly for use if symptoms recur. In pregnant women or if breastfeeding, intravaginal clotrimazole is recommended for both initial and maintenance treatment. There is little evidence on the effectiveness of natural remedies. The patient should then be reviewed in 6 months or sooner if indicated. If there are vulval symptoms, use of topical imidazoline (like Clotrimazole 1% or 2% cream applied 2–3 times a day) together with oral or intravaginal antifungal is an option.[2]

Vulvovaginal candidiasis is rare in prepubertal girls, therefore it is important to seek specialist advice for girls with recurrent infection. It is not recommended to routinely treat asymptomatic sexual partners.

KEY POINTS

- Recurrent thrush is presentation with four or more episodes in 1 year with at least partial resolution of symptoms between occurrences

- A white 'cottage cheese' discharge is commonly seen

- Microscopy, culture and sensitivity on vaginal swabs should be performed on the specimen

- Management involves advice on conservative measures

- Treatment includes an initial treatment regime for up to 14 days, followed by maintenance treatment for 6 months

References

1. Newson, L. (2010). The basics: Recurrent vaginal candidiasis. *GPOnline*, 28 May. Available at: https://www.gponline.com/basics-recurrent-vaginal-candidiasis/genito-urinary-system/article/1004744 (Accessed 4 March 2021).
2. NICE CKS. (2017). Scenario: Recurrent infection. *NICE CKS*, May. Available at: https://cks.nice.org.uk/topics/candida-female-genital/management/recurrent-infection/ (Accessed 4 March 2021).

Herpes Simplex Virus

SAI GNANASAMBANTHAN • SHREELATA DATTA

Case

An 18-year-old woman presented with a painful blister on the chin, suggestive of herpes infection. Topical acyclovir and oral antibiotic treatment were initiated. A week later, she returned with vulval pain associated with multiple ulcers and bilateral inguinal palpable lymph nodes. Polymerase chain reaction results for the fluid from the genital ulcer was positive for herpes simplex virus type 1 (HSV-1). As the patient had no history of sexual activity, the primary facial HSV-1 infection was considered most likely to have spread to the genital area via autotransmission. She was commenced on 400 mg oral acyclovir three times a day for 5 days.

Introduction and epidemiology

Herpes is very common and can be caused by both herpes simplex viruses type 1 (HSV-1) or type 2 (HSV-2). HSV-1 causes mouth ulcerations or 'cold sores' and can also be transmitted to the genitals through oral and genital sexual intercourse. HSV-2 is most often passed by vaginal and anal sexual intercourse. Some 40% of genital herpes is caused by HSV-1, whereas 22% of sexually active adults have genital herpes caused by HSV-2. HSV-1 affects the oral mucous membranes, whereas HSV-1 and 2 can affect the genitals, pubic area, buttocks and back or inner thighs. A person with herpes is not always infectious. If there are no symptoms, they are usually not infectious. The infection is only passed through direct skin-to-skin contact.

Approximately 80% of people infected with HSV-2 will have at least one recurrence, whereas only 50% of patient with HSV-1 on their genitals will have a recurrence. HSV-2 recurs on average four to six times a year, whereas HSV-1 recurs less often. Causes of recurrence can be physical (lowered immune system or local trauma) and psychologic (stress and anxiety).

Data from the United States suggests that about 2% of women are diagnosed with genital HSV infection in pregnancy. Disseminated herpes (which may present with encephalitis, hepatitis and disseminated skin lesions) is rare in adults but is commonly reported in pregnancy. Risk factors include immunocompromised mothers, such as those coinfected with human immunodeficiency virus, and smokers. Neonatal herpes has a high morbidity and mortality rate, Disseminated disease carries the worst prognosis even with antiviral treatment, with a mortality rate of 30%.[1,2]

Clinical presentation: signs and symptoms

About 80% of patients with genital herpes are unaware of the infections, as they have no symptoms or the symptoms are very mild. Of the 20% that do experience symptoms, the first indication of the infection begins between 2 and 20 days after exposure.

The symptoms start with tingling, itching, burning or pain followed by the appearance of painful red spots, which evolve within 2 days to whitish-yellow fluid-filled blisters. These then burst leaving tender ulcers, which dry and scab over. The cluster can heal in approximately 10 days. In first episodes, lesions are usually bilateral with bilateral lymphadenitis. In recurrent disease, lesions occur on favoured unilateral sites.[1] Some women may also complain of vaginal discharge and dysuria, as well as generalized fever, aches and pains, and a depressed feeling.

Some women have nonsymptomatic herpes recurrences. However, those with symptoms experience a shorter and less severe recurring episode compared with the primary occurrence.

Investigations

All women suspected to have genital herpes infection, including pregnant women, should be referred to a genitourinary medicine physician. Accurate diagnosis of genital herpes includes a thorough history and physical examination. Routine sexual health screening and smear tests do not test for herpes. Tests can only be carried out if the patient presents with symptoms and a swab is taken directly from a lesion or fluid from the blisters. The diagnosis if made by viral polymerase chain reaction. As it is possible the patient may also have contracted another sexually transmitted infection, full sexual screening should be undertaken.

Management

Once a diagnosis of herpes has been made, patients need to be encouraged to tell their partner. When blisters are present, nongenital forms of sexual contact need to be considered. Recommended regimes include acyclovir 400 mg three times daily and valaciclovir 500 mg twice daily, both for 5 days. General advice to ease symptoms includes saline baths, petroleum jelly use over the affected area, oral analgesia and 5% lidocaine topical ointment over the symptomatic area. For people who experience frequent recurrence, suppressive antiviral therapy can be used (acyclovir), which can reduce the risk of transmission as well as frequency of recurrence. Recommended regimes include acyclovir 400 mg twice daily and valaciclovir 500 mg once daily for 1 year, after which recurrence frequency should be reassessed.

Systemic infection may occur with or without widespread cutaneous lesions. The mortality from disseminated HSV is high, so early recognition and prompt treatment with intravenous antiviral treatment is essential.[1]

Pregnant women with primary genital herpes in their first or second trimester need to be advised that there is no evidence of increased risk of spontaneous miscarriage. Other risks in pregnancy include developing disseminated disease and transmission to baby during delivery and subsequently causing neonatal herpes. Management involves the use of oral or intravenous acyclovir, 400 mg three times daily or 5 days (should be used with caution before 20 weeks' gestation). It is safe and well tolerated in pregnancy. Paracetamol and topical lidocaine 2% gel can be given for symptomatic relief. As long as delivery does not occur in the next 6 weeks, the pregnancy can be managed expectantly, and vaginal delivery can be planned. However, this should be decided by the patient's obstetrician. Daily suppressive acyclovir from 36 weeks can reduce HSV lesions at term and, consequently, the need for caesarean delivery, but there is not a great deal of evidence for this. Caesarean section is usually advised for those presenting with primary herpes within 6 weeks of delivery. If the woman wants to have a vaginal delivery, rupture of membranes and invasive procedures are avoided and intravenous acyclovir intrapartum needs to be considered. Women who opt for this method also need to be advised that the risk of transmission is 41%.

With recurrent genital HSV, antiviral treatment is rarely indicated. An episode in the antenatal period is not an indication for delivery. Daily suppressive acyclovir should be used from 36 weeks to reduce the chance of lesions at the time of delivery. Women should be advised that the risk of transmission to baby is

0% to 3%. Although the risk is very low and caesarean section is not indicated, the woman should be given her options and decide on her preferred mode of delivery. When aiming for a vaginal delivery, if rupture of membranes has occurred, delivery should be expedited.[2]

KEY POINTS

- Herpes simplex virus type 1 (HSV-1) affects both oral and genital mucous membranes, whereas HSV-2 only affects genital area

- Only 20% of patients experience symptoms

- Diagnosis is made by vial polymerase chain reaction of the fluid from blisters

- Acyclovir is the treatment of choice in women, including pregnant women

- In recurrent herpes, the transmission of the virus to neonate on delivery is 0% to 3%

References

1. Patel R. (2015). 2014 UK national guideline for the management of anogenital herpes. *BASHH Guidelines*, 9 April. Available at: https://www.bashhguidelines.org/media/1019/hsv_2014-ijstda.pdf (Accessed 4 March 2021).
2. Foley E. (2014). Management of genital herpes in pregnancy. *BASHH & RCOG Guidelines*, October. Available at: https://www.rcog.org.uk/globalassets/documents/guidelines/management-genital-herpes.pdf (Accessed 4 March 2021).

Lichen Sclerosus

SAI GNANASAMBANTHAN • SHREELATA DATTA

Case

A 65-year-old woman was referred to the general gynaecology clinic by her general practitioner, with a 6-month history of vulval pruritis and dysuria. She had been treated with vaginal oestrogen cream without relief. She had a medical history of diabetes, treated with metformin. On examination, there was a lichenified plaque on the external aspect of the left labia majorum, hyperkeratosis at the introitus with fissures visible at the perineal body. Histologic findings from biopsy of the vaginal wall confirmed a diagnosis of lichen sclerosus. She was prescribed topical clobetasol 0.05% (once a night for 4 weeks, alternate nights for 4 weeks and then twice weekly for 4 weeks) and advised to apply oestrogen cream twice a week. Three months later a review showed improvement of hyperkeratosis and the patient's symptoms.

Introduction and epidemiology

Lichen sclerosus is a chronic inflammatory skin condition most often affecting the anogenital area. The pathophysiology of the condition is not fully understood, but it is often associated with autoimmune diseases, such as diabetes. Therefore it is assumed that the body's own immune system attacks the skin cells involved, resulting in the condition and its associated symptoms and signs. It is not infectious, and is therefore not sexually transmitted.[1]

The condition is a common but underdiagnosed disease that can present in either sex. However, it is more frequently seen in women than men, with a ratio ranging between 3:1 to 10:1. It is diagnosed in women of any age; however, its incidence increases with age. The prevalence in prepubertal girls is 0.1% compared with 3% in postmenopausal women.[2] Although rare, it can also be diagnosed in men.

Clinical presentation: signs and symptoms

Many patients report no symptoms, but the most common symptom of lichen sclerosus is itch. If present on nongenital skin surface, the areas seldom itch, but if present on the genital area, itching is common and can become a sore if the skin breaks down or cracks. Whilst it can heal well, the skin can scar and tighten, which can interfere with sexual intercourse, and can even constrict the urinary outflow tract.

The characteristic appearance of lichen sclerosus consists of ivory-coloured and slightly raised lesions, typically seen in the vulval or perianal regions. Other flexor surfaces, such as the back of the knee or elbows, may also be affected. After some time, the area can look like wrinkled tissue paper. The fragility of the affected area in the anogenital region can lead to bruising and erosions. The inner aspects of the labia majora and minora can eventually shrink, leading to fusion at the clitoral hood and superficial dyspareunia.

Investigations

Diagnosis can initially be clinical from observation alone. Symptoms during sexual intercourse and passing urine need to be explored. If there is any doubt of the diagnosis, or if there is no improvement using simple steroid creams, a simple skin biopsy with local anaesthetic and microscopic examination can confirm the histologic diagnosis. This may be completed in the general practice if resources are available, or in a general gynaecology clinic if more appropriate.

Management

Unfortunately, treatment is not always curative, and the symptoms may wax and wane with time. Topical steroid cream (clobetasol 0.05%) is the treatment of choice, up to three times a day for acute exacerbations, to help improve symptoms and can be used regularly for a few months. If the symptoms keep returning, the cream can be used again. In postmenopausal women, topical oestrogen cream may also help. Advice to help stop the skin becoming irritated includes washing with emollient soap substitutes, gently dabbing the area dry after passing urine, regular application of barrier cream to affected areas, using vaginal lubricant during sexual intercourse and wearing cotton or silk underwear. Things to avoid include scratching or rubbing the affected area, wearing tight or restrictive clothes and washing underwear with detergent rather than just water. Rarely, dilator therapy or surgery may be required to widen any vaginal narrowing that causes symptoms.[3]

The risk of developing genital squamous cell carcinoma in patients with lichen sclerosus over a lifetime is 4% to 5%. Therefore patients with the condition need to be reviewed in the general practice or gynaecology clinic yearly to assess for signs of cancer developing. Patient should be educated on signs to look out for, such as lumps or ulcers that do not regress.

KEY POINTS

- Lichen sclerosus is a chronic inflammatory condition associated with autoimmune disease

- It is more common in menopausal women

- The most common presenting symptom is itch

- Diagnosis is initially clinical but can be confirmed with a small biopsy

- The treatment of choice is topical steroid cream

References

1. British Skin Foundation (2002). Lichen sclerosus (in females). *Know Your Skin*. 10 June. Available at: https://knowyourskin.britishskinfoundation.org.uk/condition/lichen-sclerosus-in-females/ (Accessed 4 March 2021).
2. Pappas-Taffer K. (2020). Lichen sclerosus. *Medscape*. 25 Sept. Available at: https://emedicine.medscape.com/article/1123316-overview (Accessed 4 March 2021).
3. NHS (2018). Lichen sclerosus. *NHS*. 1 June. Available at: https://www.nhs.uk/conditions/lichen-sclerosus/#symptoms (Accessed 5 March 2021).

Lichen Planus

SAI GNANASAMBANTHAN • SHREELATA DATTA

Case

A 65-year-old Caucasian woman was referred with a 2-year history of vulval and vaginal soreness. Vulval steroid ointment and vaginal oestrogen had failed to alleviate symptoms.

On further questioning, her main complaint was superficial dyspareunia. Other complaints were dysuria and oral inflammation and ulceration.

The patient has no relevant personal or family history and was on no medication. Sexually transmitted disease and autoimmune screens were negative. The examination revealed no obvious oral ulceration and a normal vulva. The vagina was very erythematous with a narrowed introitus and thin, filmy adhesions. The examination was painful. The patient was scheduled for an examination under anaesthesia, division of vaginal adhesions and biopsies, which confirmed the diagnosis of lichen planus.

The patient was discharged on 30 mg oral prednisone daily for 7 days, with a tapering regime of 20 mg for a further 7 days and then 10 mg for the last week. Intravaginal colifoam use was also prescribed for nightly use. With support from a nurse specialist, she commenced vaginal dilator use.

Introduction and epidemiology

Lichen planus is a fairly common inflammatory rash which affects 0.2% to 1% of the population worldwide. This non-infectious condition usually occurs in adults over 40 years of age, and in women during the peri- or postmenopausal period. It occurs equally in men and women, and whilst it is not inherited, the condition can run in families.[1] Although the condition is not fully understood, an autoimmune process is thought to lead to the condition. In women with erosive genital lichen planus, 50% will give a personal or family history of an autoimmune disorder and have a 3% to 5% risk of malignant change. Commonly, it affects the skin; however, in some people it also presents on the genital area, nails, hair and mucous membranes. Of the 1% of the population who have oral lichen planus, 25% are estimated to have vulvovaginal disease. However, the genital condition is not well reported, as it is either underrecognised or asymptomatic.[2,3] In some cases, patients present with an overlap with lichen sclerosus. The signs of symptoms of the disease can also be hard to differentiate from lichen sclerosus (see Chapter 3).

Clinical presentation: signs and symptoms

The rash typically appears as small red or purple papules that are usually shiny and flat topped. They can vary in size and number. Sometimes white streaks or Wickham's striae can appear on the top of each bump. In the vulva and vagina, the rash appears as dusky pink, poorly demarcated papules with painless white streaks. The rash can develop into erythematous, sore areas. This can cause dyspareunia and scarring, which in turn can lead to narrowing of the vaginal entrance. In erosive lichen planus, painful, deep, erythematous lesions occur that overtime cause resorption of the labial structure, which is very friable. This leads to increased vaginal discharge, burning, pruritis and dyspareunia.[2]

The symptoms of itch can range from mild to very severe. When severe, it can disturb sleep and worsen the patient's quality of life.

Erosive lichen planus usually presents with erosions or glazing at the vaginal introitus that are typically edged by a lacy-white border. These lesions often persist.

Investigations

Usually the rash can be diagnosed clinically in the community. However, if there is any doubt, a biopsy can be completed under local anaesthetic in the general practice, if resources suffice, or in the general gynaecology clinic.

Management

The prognosis for erosive genital lichen planus is poor, and even with treatment, control of symptoms is difficult. Treatment should be aimed at reducing acute symptoms as you would for simple lichen planus and then maintenance with once- or twice-weekly

Dermovate ointment (0.1%) (30 g should last for more than 6 months) with follow-up in the community annually.

With treatment of simple lichen planus, the condition usually clears in 18 months and usually does not recur; however, some patients may have a second episode. Potent steroids, like 0.1% Betnovate cream or Dermovate cream once a day for 2 weeks or until lesions and symptoms improve, are used to treat repeated episodes. As symptoms improve, the frequency of topical steroids can be reduced to every other day or twice weekly. To minimise side effects of topical steroids, it is important to advise patients to treat only the itchy active lesions. A conservative approach of no treatment is an option if symptoms are mild.[3]

Antihistamines at night are an option to help ease the itch and help patients who are having particular difficulty sleeping at night. The use of topical lidocaine 2% is also an option. Emollients are helpful in providing moisture to the area and reducing the itch. A topical steroid cream is commonly used to reduce inflammation and ease the itch. However, the effect is variable and may not actually clear the rash. Steroid tablets may be considered if the rash is severe.

Where scarring of the genital area has caused narrowing, vaginal dilators coated with oestrogen or steroid cream can be advised. If this does not improve the narrowing, surgery can be considered.

The association between vulval malignancy and lichen planus has been reported in patients with erosive lichen planus; however, as it is extremely rare, the incidence is not known.[2]

KEY POINTS

- Lichen planus is an inflammatory condition commonly affecting the skin, but also other areas

- It affects both men and women equally

- Symptoms can range from mild to severe (erosive)

- Investigations involve a biopsy if a clinical diagnosis is not possible

- Several methods of treatment can be used to improve symptoms

References

1. Broadman L. (2013). Vulvovaginal disorders: Lichen planus. *Clinical Advisor*. Available at: https://www.clinicaladvisor.com/home/decision-support-in-medicine/obstetrics-and-gynecology/vulvovaginal-disorders-lichen-planus/ (Accessed 5 March 2021).

2. Starr O. (2017). Lichen planus. *Patient*. 5 Oct. Available at: https://patient.info/skin-conditions/skin-rashes/lichen-planus (Accessed 5 March 2021).
3. Edwards S. (2014). '2014 UK national guidelines on the management of vulval conditions.' *BASHH Guidelines*. 8 Oct. Available at: https://www.bashhguidelines.org/media/1056/vulval-conditions_2014-ijstda.pdf (Accessed 5 March 2021).

Genital Warts

SAI GNANASAMBANTHAN • SHREELATA DATTA

Case

A 34-year-old woman presented requesting an examination, as her current sexual partner had divulged that he had previously been diagnosed with genital warts and recently had a recurrence. She uses the oral contraceptive for birth control. Her last smear test result was normal 6 months ago, with no previous abnormal results. Examination of her genitalia revealed multiple small (<0.5 cm), flesh-coloured raised papules in the perineal area. She opted for topical Podoflox 0.5% gel therapy, twice daily for 3 days and then weekly until the lesions and symptoms resolve. At her follow-up appointment 3 weeks later, the lesions had subsided, and the patient complained of no further symptoms.

Introduction and epidemiology

Genital warts is the most commonly diagnosed viral sexually transmitted infection (STI), accounting for 15.7% of all STI diagnoses in 2015. The condition is sometimes referred to as condyloma acuminata or venereal warts. The condition is caused by the human papilloma virus (HPV). There are over 100 types of the virus, of which 40 can infect the genital and anal areas in both men and women. High-risk strains are linked to virtually all cervical cancers, but can also cause vaginal, vulval, penile and anal cancer, whereas low-risk types (6 and 11) are associated with 75% to 100% of genital wart cases. It has a global prevalence of 10.4%, most commonly presenting in patients under the age of 30 years; the prevalence decreases rapidly with age. The incubation period can vary, with warts developing from within a month of acquiring the virus to years. Some people can carry the virus but not develop any warts. The peak incidence of the disease occurs during 16 to 25 years of age. Key risk factors include intercourse at an early age, number of lifetime sexual partners and immunosuppressive disorders such as human immunodeficiency virus.[1]

Clinical presentation: signs and symptoms

Genital warts usually present as small, fleshy growths anywhere on the external genitalia. They can vary in shape, size and number. Although painless, they can be bothersome because of their location, size or itching. Associated discharge may also be present. Rarely urinary outflow obstruction may occur, or the warts may bleed. In women, they usually occur on the labia minora or vaginal introitus. Lesions visible on the outer genital mucosa require a thorough examination of the vaginal canal, cervix and anorectal areas. Bleeding or pain during intercourse is rare.

Investigations

Diagnosis is often made by a thorough history and examination of the patient. Sometimes lesions are not so obvious and may require acetowhitening enhanced technique, with the application of 5% acetic acid to the area in question, and a diagnosis is made if the lesions turn white. Colposcopy may also be necessary to look at lesions in the canal and cervix. A biopsy can be performed if the lesions appear suspicious or recur after treatment. A routine smear test will also check for HPV if abnormal cells are found on cytology because of the high association between HPV infection and cervical cancer.

Management

Treatment includes topical applications (Podophyllotoxin, Imiquimod and trichloroacetic acid) and physical ablation (cryotherapy, electrosurgery, excision and laser). Podophyllotoxin is a first-line treatment, available as a 0.5% solution or 0.15% cream and self-applied twice daily for 3 days and repeated weekly. It is not recommended in pregnancy. Trichloroacetic acid results in tissue necrosis and therefore should be applied weekly in clinic and not appropriate for-large volume warts. Imiquimod 5% cream three times a week has a 10% recurrence rate by 3 months.

Cryotherapy in the form of liquid nitrogen spray or probe or a nitrous oxide probe can be used once weekly. It is safe in pregnancy. Electrocautery, excision or laser ablation is completed in a single visit and requires local anaesthetic. Recurrence rates range from 3% to 77%.[2]

Because no treatment is 100% effective, the focus has moved to preventing HPV infection. In the United Kingdom, the HPV vaccine Gardasil is currently advised for girls aged 12 to 18 years. However, it is currently only available for women and is not given to men. It is effective in preventing HPV infection with subtypes 6, 11, 16 and 18 in women who have had no previous infection. However, it is less effective in patients who have already been infected and of course does not protect against all strains. Gardasil 9 is effective against the four common strains of HPV, as well as subtypes 31, 33, 45, 52 and 58. In England, girls aged 12 to 13 years are offered the first vaccine at school, and the second dose is offered 6 to 12 months after this. Once infected, the HPV stays in the human body as an active infection (which can be transmitted), lays dormant or, in 9 out 10 cases, is cleared away within 2 years.

KEY POINTS

- Genital warts is the most commonly diagnosed sexually transmitted infection and is caused by human papilloma virus (HPV)

- They are caused by low-risk strains 6 and 11

- They occur commonly in the anogenital areas

- Treatment is either topical or physical ablation

- Gardasil vaccine was developed to prevent the spread of HPV because of the difficulty in treating the condition

References

1. Gilson R. (2015). UK national guidelines on the management of anogenital warts 2015. *BASHH guidelines*. April. Available at: https://www.bashhguidelines.org/media/1075/uk-national-guideline-on-warts-2015-final.pdf (Accessed 5 March 2021).
2. Stoppler M. (2019). Genital herpes. *Emedicinehealth*. 10 March. Available at: https://www.emedicinehealth.com/genital_herpes/article_em.htm (Accessed 5 March 2021).

The Immunocompromised Patient with Genitourinary Presentations

SAI GNANASAMBANTHAN • SHREELATA DATTA

Case

A 30-year-old nurse was diagnosed with human immunodeficiency virus (HIV) 6 months ago following investigation of a needle-stick injury. She presented to the Genitourinary clinic complaining of a genital ulcer and rash over both hands and feet, which was noted 6 days ago. She gave a history of unprotected sexual intercourse with her new partner for the last month.

On examination, she was afebrile with bilateral cervical lymphadenopathy and a maculopapular rash over her palms and soles of her feet. Also noted was a small ulcer or chancre on her right labia.

Swabs of the ulcer confirmed syphilis, with blood immunoglobulin (Ig)M results also being positive. She was given Benzathine penicillin G 2.4 mega units as a single dose intramuscularly.

Introduction and epidemiology

Women living with HIV in the United Kingdom need adequate support and access to services that enable them to have the best sexual health, while also avoiding transmission of HIV and all sexually transmitted infections (STIs). In 2005 it was noted that 63% of HIV infections acquired through heterosexual contact were in women in the United Kingdom. Some 64% of women diagnosed with HIV were 25 to 39 years of age and therefore sexually active, hence the need for regular STI assessments. The management of most STI infections in HIV women does not differ from the treatment of those without HIV. However, manifestation of symptoms of certain STIs can be more severe and rapidly progressive.

Herpes simplex infection activates HIV replication and increases HIV transmission. It is the most common STI in HIV-positive heterosexual patients in the United Kingdom.[1] The amount of

HIV-associated immunosuppression is the main risk factor for HSV reactivation. Syphilis is mostly seen in Caucasian homosexual men aged 25 to 34 years old, 40% of whom are coinfected with HIV.

Clinical presentation: signs and symptoms

Presentation of STIs is similar in HIV patients compared with patients without the disease. However, severity can be worse when immunocompromised, as well as have an increased risk of recurrence and quick progression of symptoms. STIs should always be considered as a differential diagnosis in HIV patients presenting with a rash.[2]

With herpes simplex virus (HSV), clinical lesions might be resistant to management and progressive in patients with HIV. Genital herpes and chronic erosive lesions occur as a symptom of immune reconstitution inflammatory syndrome (IRIS) as a result of a mix of antiretroviral medications.[1]

Primary syphilis in a HIV-negative patient presents with a single papule and moderate regional lymphadenopathy. The papule then ulcerates and is painless but indurated. In the context of HIV coinfections, there may be multiple, painless ulcers that are deeper and can persist into the secondary stage of the infection. The bacteria disseminates widely early on via blood and lymphatics. The secondary stage does not have mucocutaneous signs like HIV-negative patients. Instead it results in hepatitis, glomerulonephritis and splenomegaly. Some 1% to 2% of patients develop neurologic symptoms during this phase.[3]

Investigations

Sexual health screening involves genital swabs for culture of gonorrhoea and chlamydia, blood and swabs from sores can be tested by polymerase chain reaction (PCR) for syphilis, and viral PCR of swabs can be completed for HSV. If oral or pharyngeal symptoms are present, these too need investigation with viral swabs for PCR. This complete sexual health screen needs to be completed and documented at the time of diagnosis of HIV patients, as well as reviewed every 6 months. Syphilis serology needs to be included in basic HIV blood tests every 3 months. Both treponemal and nontreponemal serology tests act the same way in HIV-positive and negative patients. However, false-negative results are more common in HIV-infected individuals. All HIV patients presenting with neurology symptoms need to have cerebrospinal fluid (CSF) PCR for neurosyphilis. CSF abnormalities consistent with neurosyphilis are commonly seen in patients with advanced HIV. Because of the high prevalence of lymphogranuloma venereum in HIV patients, they should all be tested and treated with 3 weeks of doxycycline if positive for Chlamydia.[1–4]

Management

The majority of STIs in HIV-positive patients can be managed in the same way as in patients without the disease. Initial syphilis serology at diagnosis of HIV needs to be documented and taken as part of the HIV blood set to rule out asymptomatic syphilis. The management of gonorrhoea, non-specific urethritis, uncomplicated Chlamydia and lymphogranuloma venereum in HIV-positive patients does not differ significantly from patients without HIV.

Patients with herpes simplex virus type 2 (HSV-2), who are also HIV positive, are prone to increased symptomatic and asymptomatic shedding. This risk is increased further if the patient has a low CD4 count and in those who test positive for HSV-1. Standard systemic antiviral drugs used in patients without HIV are effective in treating genital herpes in HIV-positive patients. However, resistance is also more common, and hence treatment failure also. Prompt treatment is recommended with double the standard dose in advanced HIV. Recommended regimes include acyclovir 400 mg five times daily for 7 to 10 days and valaciclovir 500 mg to 1 g twice daily for 10 days. Treatment should be continued till all lesions have re-epithelialised. In severe cases, acyclovir 5 to 10 mg/kg body weight intravenously three times daily may be required for 2 to 7 days or until clinical improvement is seen. This should be followed by oral therapy to complete a minimum of 10 days total. Suppressive antiviral therapy (acyclovir 400 mg twice daily or valaciclovir 500 mg once daily orally) can be considered to help prevent viral shedding and also reduce genital HIV shedding. Management of erosive lesions and herpes caused by IRIS in HIV-positive patients is difficult to manage but may respond to topical cidofovir.[1]

Most guidelines recommend the same treatment protocol for syphilis in HIV-positive and HIV-negative patients. HIV-positive patients may, however, be at increased risk of treatment failure. Patients with neurosyphilis need to be treated with 2.4 g of procaine penicillin once daily intramuscularly for 10 to 14 days, plus probenecid 500 mg orally four times daily for the same duration. No other treatment regime has been proven more effective in preventing neurosyphilis in HIV patients.[3]

All HIV-positive patients require a sexual health assessment, including a thorough history, documented when they are first diagnosed. Assessments need to be regularly carried out at 6-month intervals after initial diagnosis. Patients should be given information on how to access sexual health clinics and require continued counselling and support to maintain good sexual health.[2]

KEY POINTS

- The management of most sexually transmitted infection (STI) in human immunodeficiency virus (HIV)-positive women does not differ from the treatment of those without HIV

- HSV is the most common STI in HIV-positive heterosexual patients in the United Kingdom

- Primary syphilis in HIV patients presents as multiple painless ulcers that are deeper and can persist into the secondary stage of the infection

- All HIV-positive patients require a sexual health assessment at first diagnosis and 6-month assessments thereafter

References

1. Patel R. (2015). 2014 UK national guideline for the management of anogenital herpes. *BASHH Guidelines*. 9 April. Available at: https://www.bashhguidelines.org/media/1019/hsv_2014-ijstda.pdf (Accessed 4 March 2021).
2. Fakoya A. (2008). British HIV Association, BASHH and FSRH guidelines for the management of the sexual and reproductive health of people living with HIV infection 2008. *BASHH Guidelines*. 2008. Available at: https://www.bashhguidelines.org/media/1068/sexual-reproductive-health.pdf (Accessed 8 March 2021).
3. Kingston M. (2015). UK national guidelines on the management of syphilis 2015. *BASHH Guidelines*. 2 Dec. Available at: https://www.bashhguidelines.org/media/1148/uk-syphilis-guidelines-2015.pdf (Accessed 8 March 2021).
4. Nwokolo N. (2015). 2015 UK national guideline for the management of infection with Chlamydia trachomatis. *BASHH Guidelines*. 9 Oct. Available at: https://www.bashhguidelines.org/media/1045/chlamydia-2015.pdf (Accessed 8 March 2021).

Intermenstrual/Postcoital Bleeding

NEKTARIA VAROUXAKI • SHREELATA DATTA

Case

A 43-year-old woman presented to her general practitioner (GP) surgery with a history of new-onset postcoital bleeding. She reported an onset of her symptoms approximately 1 week prior after every episode of intercourse. She describes small amounts of fresh bleeding per vagina lasting 24 hours. Her last smear was 6 months ago and was normal. She does not have a history of abnormal smears. She is not complaining of any other symptoms and she is otherwise fit and well. On examination, the abdomen was soft, non-tender and non-distended. On speculum examination, the GP noted an endocervical polyp protruding through the os. Vulva and vagina appeared healthy, and bimanual examination was essentially normal. She was referred to the gynaecology outpatient department, where the findings were confirmed and she was added to the waiting list for polypectomy. A transvaginal scan was also requested which revealed, normal uterus, endometrial lining and ovaries.

Introduction and epidemiology

Intermenstrual bleeding is defined as any bleeding which occurs outside of the woman's menstrual period, and it also includes postcoital bleeding. It affects approximately 13% to 21% of women and 24% of perimenopausal women. Some 3% to 18% of women presenting with postcoital bleeding have cervical intraepithelial neoplasia or cervical cancer.[2] Causes of postcoital/intermenstrual bleeding are presented in Table 7.1.

Clinical presentation: signs and symptoms

The signs and symptoms depend on the cause. For example, if the cause is infective (e.g. chlamydia), the woman may also complain

Table 7.1

Causes of Postcoital/Intermenstrual Bleeding[2]	
Causes	
Ovarian	Ovulation (1%–2% of women)
	Oestrogen-secreting tumours
Uterine	Iatrogenic (hormonal contraception, anticoagulants)
	Infective (endometritis)
	Structural benign (polyps, fibroids, adenomyosis)
	Structural malignant (endometrial cancer)
Cervical	Iatrogenic (postexamination/smear)
	Infective (chlamydia/gonorrhoea)
	Structural benign (ectropion, polyps)
	Structural malignant (cervical cancer)
Vaginal	Infective (trichomonas vaginalis, candida albicans)
	Structural benign (vaginal adenosis)
	Structural malignant (vaginal cancer)

of offensive vaginal discharge, dysuria, dyspareunia or abdominal pain. Therefore thorough clinical history and examination are important to identify possible causes of intermenstrual/postcoital bleeding. The importance of obtaining a clear smear history cannot be stressed enough.

Investigations

Cervical smear (only if the woman is due one) as well as high vaginal and endocervical swabs (to rule out infective causes) are usually needed. A transvaginal scan will rule out most ovarian and uterine causes. The woman should be referred for colposcopy if there is an obvious cervical lesion/abnormality or if the woman is complaining of persistent postcoital bleeding or vaginal discharge despite normal cervical cytology and swabs.[3] Pregnancy should also always be ruled out.

Management

Management is guided by the possible cause. For example, appropriate antibiotics/antifungals will treat infective causes, whereas changing the dosage/type of hormone used will treat intermenstrual/postcoital bleeding attributed to hormonal contraception. Malignant causes should be investigated and managed according to local and national protocols.

KEY POINTS

- Intermenstrual/postcoital bleeding is a common symptom, especially during perimenopause

- Cervical pathology should always be ruled out in women presenting with postcoital bleeding

- Cervical cytology should be obtained only if the woman is due a smear according to the national screening programme (every 3 years for women aged 25–49 years and every 5 years for women 49–64 years)

- Investigations and management are decided according to possible causes

References

1. https://elearning.rcog.org.uk/.
2. Wan, Y. L., Edmondson, R. J., & Crosbie, E. J. (2015). Intermenstrual and postcoital bleeding. Obstetrics, Gynaecology & Reproductive Medicine, 2015;25:106-112.
3. NHS Cervical Screening Programme. Colposcopy and Programme Management. Guidelines for the NHS Cervical Screening Programme. 3rd Ed. NHSCSP Publication No 20. Sheffield:NHSCSP;2016.

Premenstrual Syndrome

SAI GNANASAMBANTHAN • SHREELATA DATTA

Case

A 30-year-old married woman presents to her general practitioner (GP) complaining that for roughly a week each month she develops irritability and mood swings, lashing out verbally at her husband and three children. She is impatient and feels overwhelmed and out of control in her reactions to stressors. She also complains of tiredness, interrupted sleep, cravings for sweets, abdominal bloating, headaches and breast tenderness during this time. The patient's symptoms increase in severity with the approach of her period but diminish and even resolve on the first day she bleeds. The patient is requesting help because of the toll it has taken on her marriage and her relationship with her children. Although she feels she is more tense and less efficient at work when she is premenstrual, her functioning on the job has not been impaired.

Her past psychiatric history includes postpartum depression 2 weeks after the birth of her first child, 8 years ago. The depression was successfully treated with a tricyclic antidepressant and supportive psychotherapy for 6 months, with full recovery. The patient also remembers her mother being very 'moody and anxious' intermittently when she was growing up. Her past medical history was unremarkable.

Her physical examination was unremarkable. She was sent for blood tests and asked to complete a diary of her symptoms with a view to reassessing her in 2 months. On return, her blood tests were normal. Her diary showed her symptoms lasted 10 days, beginning 10 days before her period and completely resolving on day 1 of her cycle. During her follicular phase she had no symptoms at all. Premenstrual syndrome (PMS) was diagnosed and discussed with the patient. Therapies were run through with efficacies. The patient wanted to try avoiding medication in the first instance because of the fear of non-compliance with three children. She was referred to cognitive behavioural therapy in the first instance.

Introduction and epidemiology

PMS is a mixture of psychologic and physical symptoms that appear during the second half or luteal phase of the menstrual cycle (up to 14 days before menstruation). The key feature of this condition is that the clinical symptoms usually disappear with the end of menstruation, and patients remain symptom-free till ovulation. Differentiating between physiologic menstrual symptoms and PMS can be difficult, so the clinician needs to take a thorough history. Detecting symptoms in association with the patient's menstrual cycle, as described earlier, together with identifying the degree of impact on their quality of life, directs the clinician to the diagnosis of PMS.

With 3% to 8% of women affected by severe PMS, and 40% of women presenting with symptoms of PMS, it is crucial that clinicians understand the disease and manage these women effectively. Two theories of the aetiology involve the ovarian hormone cycle, strengthened by the fact that PMS is absent before puberty, during pregnancy, and after the menopause, and during treatment with gonadotrophin-releasing hormone (GnRH) analogues. Existing theories are based on the idea that some women are particularly sensitive to progesterone and progestogens (progesterone levels are similar in women with or without PMS), or that serotonin plays a role, as oestrogen and progesterone affect serotonin levels and selective serotonin reuptake inhibitors (SSRIs) reduce PMS symptoms.[1,2]

Clinical presentation: signs and symptoms

Each woman's symptoms are different and can also vary between each cycle.

The most common symptoms of PMS include:

- mood swings
- feeling upset, anxious or irritable
- tiredness or trouble sleeping
- bloating or abdominal pain
- breast tenderness
- headaches
- skin changes (for example, spots)
- changes in appetite
- changes in sex drive[1]

Investigations

A diary of symptoms over two menstrual cycles is required to aid the diagnosis of PMS. A thorough history is essential when seeing these patients, and when prospective symptoms appear during the luteal phase and resolve during or at the end of menstruation, diagnosis is reinforced. Several tools can be used to help clinicians assess the severity of symptoms and reach a diagnosis.[1] The Daily Record of Severity of Problems (shown in Box 8.1) is one such tool that has proven to be valuable to health professionals and is well validated. Patients score symptoms each day using a 6-point scale (1 = not at all, 2 = minimal, 3 = mild, 4 = moderate, 5 = severe, 6 = extreme). The scores are added in the column for the first day of menses. A total of less than 50 excludes PMS as a diagnosis. When a total score of greater than 50 is reported, the same report is run for the next cycle. If more than three items have an average score of more than 3 during the luteal phase, the scores of 5-day

---

Box 8.1 Daily Record of Severity of Problems

- 1a Felt depressed, sad, 'down' or 'blue'
- 1b Felt hopeless
- 1c Felt worthless, or guilty
- 2 Felt anxious, tense, 'keyed up' or 'on edge'
- 3a Had mood swings (e.g. suddenly felt sad or tearful)
- 3b Was more sensitive to rejection or feelings were easily hurt
- 4a Felt angry, irritable
- 4b Had conflicts or problems with people
- 5 Had less interest in usual activities (e.g. work, school, friends, hobbies)
- 6 Had difficulty concentrating
- 7 Felt lethargic, tired, fatigued or had a lack of energy
- 8a Had increased appetite or overate
- 8b Had cravings for specific foods
- 9a Slept more, took naps, found it hard to get up when intended
- 9b Had trouble getting to sleep or staying asleep
- 10a Felt overwhelmed or unable to cope
- 10b Felt out of control
- 11a Had breast tenderness
- 11b Had breast swelling, felt 'bloated' or had weight gain
- 11c Had headache
- 11d Had joint or muscle pain
- At work, at school, at home, or in daily routine, at least one of the problems noted earlier caused reduction in productivity or inefficiency
- At least one of the problems noted earlier interfered with hobbies or social activities (e.g. avoid or do less)
- At least one of the problems noted earlier interfered with relationships with others

intervals during the luteal and follicular phases are added. A luteal phase score, 30% greater than the follicular phase score signposts PMS. Sometimes, a third cycle of a symptom diary is needed if the diagnosis remains unclear. Other tools, such as the Premenstrual Symptoms Screening Tool and various new phone apps, are all easily accessible but not validated to diagnose the condition.

If symptom diaries provide confusing results, GnRH analogues (inhibits cyclical ovarian function) can be used for a 3-month period, to differentiate those with and without PMS, aiding diagnosis. The first month allows the agonist to suppress the hormone effect, followed by two further months to keep a symptom diary.

Management

As primary clinicians, GPs are at the forefront of seeing these women, therefore awareness of the disease and ability to manage appropriately are essential. Secondary care professionals such as a gynaecologist or a psychiatrist should be sought when simple measures implemented by GPs have failed, symptom diaries are inconclusive, or an underlying psychiatric or somatic disorder is apparent, that is. A multidisciplinary team can implement a unique patient care plan using a variety of treatments in the specialist setting.

Management is implemented and escalated in a stepwise manner. Clinicians can consider starting with non-pharmacologic treatment (including discussion of complementary therapies), proceeding to antidepressant and hormonal medications, and considering surgical options as a last resort.

Non-pharmacologic therapy

Evidence regarding the effectiveness of complementary therapies is limited, but they can be considered for women where hormonal treatments are contraindicated. Table 8.1 outlines the current available holistic therapies and the evidence of benefit to patients suffering with PMS symptoms. The evidence of benefit when suggesting these options should always be discussed with the patient, highlighting that there is little conclusive evidence to support their use.

A systematic review showed evidence of calcium alleviating physical and psychologic symptoms in PMS. When considering St John's Wort, be aware that it interacts with other medications, such as SSRIs, and can make low-dose combined oral contraceptives ineffective.

In mild PMS, cognitive behavioural therapy to help with relaxation methods, stress management and assertiveness training can be effective. If useful in alleviating symptoms, patients could avoid

Table 8.1

Summarises Current Research Into the Benefits of Selected Complementary Therapies for the Treatment of Premenstrual Syndrome[1]	
Complementary therapy	**Benefit**
Exercise	Some benefit
Reflexology	Some benefit
Vitamin B6	Mixed results
Magnesium	Mixed results
Multivitamins	Unknown
Calcium/vitamin D	Yes
Isoflavones	Mixed results
Vitex agnus castus L	Yes – Inadequate safety data
St John's Wort	Mixed results
Ginkgo biloba	Some benefit
Saffron	Yes
Evening primrose oil	Some benefit
Acupuncture	Some benefit
Lemon balm	Some benefit
Curcumin	Some benefit
Wheat germ	Some benefit

pharmacotherapy and potential side effects. However, this method has a slower response compared with SSRIs, but better maintenance.

Hormonal treatment

In hormonal treatment, newer combined contraceptives with antimineralocorticoid and antiandrogenic progestogens are shown to suppress ovulation, without generating progestogen-related PMS symptoms. Examples include Drospirenone 3 mg once a day and Ethinyl oestradiol 20 mcg once a day. It should be used as first-line therapy (if not contraindicated in the patient), especially if the patient requires contraception as well. It is also suggested that continuous therapy has a better effect on mood, headache and pelvic pain scores, compared with cyclical therapy.

Oestrogen therapy is another option for inhibiting ovulation in PMS. Transdermal patches are preferred to the implant. However, progesterone opposition to the oestrogen is needed to prevent endometrial hyperplasia, unless the patient has had a hysterectomy. The lowest dose for the shortest time (micronized progesterone, 100 or 200 mg, once a day) should be used to prevent progestogen-induced PMS symptoms. Alternatively, use of the levonorgestrel-releasing intrauterine system (LNG-IUS, to directly work on the endometrium) can reduce recurrence of progesterone-induced PMS symptoms. Patients should always be advised that at first, PMS-like symptoms may still occur. The treatment combinations suggested include percutaneous oestradiol and either a cyclical 10- to 12-day course of oral or vaginal progesterone or LNG-IUS 52 mg. There should be a low threshold for investigating unscheduled bleeding when low doses of progesterone are used. Women should also be advised that there is little evidence on the long-term effects on the endometrium and breast tissue when using oestradiol treatments.

Long-acting GnRH analogues are also effective in treating severe PMS. They work by suppressing ovarian functioning and therefore inhibiting the menstrual cycle. Although in the long term this is a good option, in the short term the treatment causes hot flashes, night sweats, low mood and insomnia, and patients should be warned about this. In the long term, the oestrogen deficiency can also cause vaginal atrophy, increased cardiovascular risk and osteoporosis, therefore treatment without add-back therapy should be limited to 6 months. If add-back therapy from 6 months is used in the long term, bone mineral density should also be assessed annually by dual-energy x-ray absorptiometry scanning. Although hormone replacement therapy (HRT) can decrease the side effects of oestrogen deficiency, it can cause PMS-like symptoms. Considering all of this, GnRH analogues should be reserved for the most severe symptoms, or if other treatments have failed. If patients fail to respond to GnRH analogues, then the PMS diagnosis should be questioned. Although not licenced, GnRH analogues are used to aid diagnosis where 2-month diaries do not reveal PMS.[1,2]

Non-hormonal treatment

In severe PMS, selective SSRIs (fluoxetine 20–60 mg, citalopram 20–40 mg and sertraline 50–150 mg) can be considered along with GnRH analogues as first-line treatment. They affect the emotional, behavioural and physical symptoms of core PMD. SSRIs work quickly, so they can be taken sequentially in the luteal phase and continuously. Patients should be aware of side effects (nausea, fatigue, insomnia and sexual dysfunction) of SSRIs, which are reduced with intermittent use, and that PMS symptoms recur when SSRIs are stopped. If administered continuously, the dose needs to be tapered off to prevent withdrawal symptoms. This is less of an issue if taken in the luteal phase alone. Women should be given accurate prepregnancy counselling and told that PMS symptoms will stop during pregnancy, so SSRIs can be discontinued. Women should be informed that there is a possible, but unproven, association with congenital malformations, so ideally they should stop SSRIs before and during pregnancy.

The use of diuretics, such as spironolactone 100 mg, may also ameliorate physical symptoms, weight gain and mood.[1,2]

Surgical treatment

Having a hysterectomy together with bilateral salpingoophorectomy, is the definitive method of ending the ovarian cycle. As the endometrium is also removed, progesterone opposition is not required when oestrogen is given. This surgical option is justified for women with debilitating symptoms in whom medical treatment has failed, where long-term GnRH analogue medication is needed, or other gynaecologic pathologies require a hysterectomy.

Preoperative GnRH analogues should be used as a 'test of cure', to ensure that HRT will be tolerated, especially in women under 45 years of age considering surgery for PMS alone. Following surgery, oestrogen-only HRT should be advised. By avoiding progestogen treatment PMS-type symptoms are avoided. Replacing testosterone is also important to maintain libido, as the ovaries produce 50% of it (Fig. 8.1).

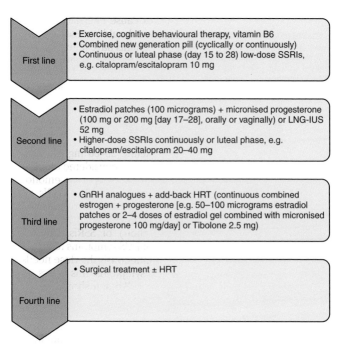

First line
- Exercise, cognitive behavioural therapy, vitamin B6
- Combined new generation pill (cyclically or continuously)
- Continuous or luteal phase (day 15 to 28) low-dose SSRIs, e.g. citalopram/escitalopram 10 mg

Second line
- Estradiol patches (100 micrograms) + micronised progesterone (100 mg or 200 mg [day 17–28], orally or vaginally) or LNG-IUS 52 mg
- Higher-dose SSRIs continuously or luteal phase, e.g. citalopram/escitalopram 20–40 mg

Third line
- GnRH analogues + add-back HRT (continuous combined estrogen + progesterone [e.g. 50–100 micrograms estradiol patches or 2–4 doses of estradiol gel combined with micronised progesterone 100 mg/day] or Tibolone 2.5 mg)

Fourth line
- Surgical treatment ± HRT

Figure 8.1 Flow chart to help with steps of management.[1,2]

KEY POINTS

- Premenstrual syndrome (PMS) is a mixture of psychologic and physical symptoms affecting women who menstruate

- The key characteristic is that clinical symptoms usually cease by the end of menstruation

- A diary of symptoms over two menstrual cycles is required to aid the diagnosis of PMS

- Management is implemented and escalated in a stepwise manner, and include non-pharmacology therapies, hormonal and non-hormonal medications, and surgery

- Discussion with patients is key in diagnosis and deciding on an appropriate treatment plan

References

1. Gnanasambanthan S, Datta S. Premenstrual syndrome. *Obstet Gynaecol Reprod Med* 2019;29(10):281-5.
2. Royal College of Obstetricians & Gynaecologists (2016).'Management of premenstrual syndrome. *Green-top Guideline No. 48. 30* Nov. Available at: https://obgyn. onlinelibrary.wiley.com/doi/full/10.1111/1471-0528.14260 (Accessed 8 March 2021).

Postmenopausal Bleeding

NEKTARIA VAROUXAKI • SHREELATA DATTA

Case

A 62-year-old woman presented to her general practitioner follow-ing an episode of postmenopausal bleeding (PMB) approximately 2 days ago. She underwent the menopause at the age of 52 years and has had no previous episodes of PMB. Her smears have always been normal and are up-to-date. The episode was not related to intercourse. Her body mass index (BMI) is 36 kg/m^2 and she is on treatment for essential hypertension and diabetes mellitus type 2. She has had four spontaneous vaginal deliveries. Her surgical history is unremarkable. There is no family history of gynaecologic malignancy.

On examination, abdomen was soft, non-tender and non-distended. Vulva, vagina and cervix appeared healthy. A small amount of blood was noted in the posterior fornix.

A transvaginal scan was requested and performed to assess the endometrial thickness. The endometrium measured 11 mm and appeared irregular; both ovaries were normal. In view of the findings, an urgent hysteroscopy and biopsy were performed. The biopsy revealed a diagnosis of endometrioid uterine adeno-carcinoma.

Introduction and epidemiology

Postmenopausal bleeding is defined as any vaginal bleeding that occurs in a woman after at least 1 year of secondary amenorrhoea. It is a symptom that is seen in approximately 4% to 11% of post-menopausal women. The most common causes of PMB are shown in Table 9.1.

One in 10 women who experience postmenopausal bleeding will be diagnosed with endometrial cancer. It is the most common pelvic gynaecologic cancer and the fourth most common cancer overall. Peak age of endometrial cancer is 65 to 75 years.[1]

Table 9.1

Most Common Causes of Postmenopausal Bleeding[2]	
Atrophic endometrium	45%
Hormone replacement therapy	20%
Endometrial polyps	15%
Endometrial cancer	10%
Endometrial hyperplasia	10%

Risk factors for endometrial cancer include:

- Unopposed oestrogen exposure which has a proliferative effect on the endometrium, which in turn causes hyperplasia and then malignancy
- Late menopause
- Nulliparity
- Obesity
- Hypertension
- Diabetes mellitus
- Hormone replacement therapy
- Polycystic ovarian syndrome
- Tamoxifen

Clinical presentation: signs and symptoms

The woman will present with vaginal bleeding after menopause (1 year or more since the last menstrual period). The woman might be also complaining of persistent vaginal discharge.

Physical examination is essential and should consist of abdominal examination, speculum examination and bimanual pelvic examination.

Investigations

PMB should be investigated under the 2-week wait rule. A transvaginal scan is needed to assess the endometrial thickness, as well as the ovaries. Systematic reviews have suggested a cut-off of 3 to 4 mm for ruling out endometrial cancer and have shown that the probability of cancer is reduced to less than 1% when the endometrial thickness is less than the cut-off.[3]

Management

If the endometrial thickness is less than the cut-off, no further action is required, unless the PMB persists/recurs. If the endometrium is thickened, then the endometrial biopsy will give a diagnosis of the cause of PMB. Regarding methods of obtaining a sample from the endometrium, this can be done by using outpatient sampling devices (Pipelle) or by hysteroscopy (inpatient or outpatient). The failure rate of outpatient sampling devices is approximately 10%. Management once diagnosis is made is defined by the cause.

KEY POINTS

- The most common cause of PMB is atrophic endometritis/vaginitis

- Endometrial cancer should always be ruled out in a postmenopausal woman who presents with PMB

- Transvaginal ultrasound to evaluate the endometrial thickness is the gold standard for investigation of PMB

- If the endometrium is thickened–that is, 4 mm or above–hysteroscopy and biopsy will give a diagnosis of the cause of PMB

References

1. https://www.cancerresearchuk.org/health-professional/cancer-statistics/statistics-by-cancer-type/uterine-cancer/incidence
2. elearning.rcog.org.uk; gynaecological oncology; malignant disease of the uterus; 2017
3. A. Timmermans et al. Endometrial thickness measurement for detecting endometrial cancer in women with postmenopausal bleeding: a systematic review and meta-analysis. *Obstet Gynecol* 2010;116:160–167.

Domestic Violence

NEKTARIA VAROUXAKI • SHREELATA DATTA

Case

A 28-year-old pregnant woman attended her general practitioner's surgery for her 28-week antenatal appointment. She had missed her 20-week anomaly scan, as well as previous antenatal appointments with her midwife. This is her fourth pregnancy, having had two termination of pregnancies and one early miscarriage at 8 weeks' gestation. She told the midwife that she was away and had not been able to reschedule her missed appointments. When the midwife tried to measure the symphysis-fundal height and auscultate the foetal heart rate, she noticed bruising on the woman's abdomen and chest. On further questioning, the woman admitted to being in an abusive relationship. She also reported non-consensual sexual intercourse. She was referred to the named midwife and was advised that she could report the case to the police, and steps were taken to secure a place in a women's refuge after she decided that she was willing to leave her partner. Psychologic support was also offered and accepted. The rest of the pregnancy was uncomplicated, and the woman had a vaginal delivery at 41 weeks.

Introduction/epidemiology

Domestic abuse is defined as abuse of one partner within an intimate or family relationship of those aged 16 years or over regardless of gender or equality. Statistics reveal that one in four women in the United Kingdom has been a victim of domestic violence and that approximately 30% of abuse commences during pregnancy. Moreover, 4% to 9% of women are abused during pregnancy and/or after delivery. There is evidence that women who are being abused are at higher risk of obstetric complications, such as placental abruption, preterm delivery, low birth weight, antepartum haemorrhage, stillbirth and perinatal mental health disorders. They also have higher rates of terminations of pregnancy.[1] Therefore every woman should be asked about abuse during pregnancy and should also have at least one consultation on her own.

In the aforementioned case, the woman is also a victim of sexual assault/rape. The World Health Organization defines sexual violence as 'any sexual act, attempt to obtain a sexual act, unwanted sexual comments or advances, or acts to traffic, or otherwise directed, against a person's sexuality using coercion, by any person regardless of their relationship to the victim, in any setting, including but not limited to home and work'.[2] The Sexual Offences Act 2003 that applies to England and Wales defines sexual assault when: '(1) a person intentionally touches another person; (2) the touching is sexual; and (3) the person does not consent'. The maximum prison sentence for this is 10 years. The Sexual Offences Act 2003 also defines a serious sexual assault as assault by penetration. This means that they intentionally penetrate the vagina or anus of another person with a part of the body or anything else, without that person's consent. This encompasses the definition of rape where penetration of the vagina, anus or mouth of a person has occurred with a penis without consent. The maximum sentence for this is life imprisonment.[3,4]

Clinical presentation

Domestic abuse includes physical, psychologic, sexual, financial and emotional abuse. Different forms of abuse commonly co-exist, just like in the earlier example. Women who are in abusive relationships often miss their antenatal appointments or, on the contrary, have multiple attendances in Accidents & Emergency/Medical Assessment Unit with different complaints (e.g. abdominal pain, reduced foetal movements etc.). Signs of abuse, such as bruising, abrasions or lacerations, can also be noticed during physical examination of the woman. Unfortunately, the majority of cases of sexual assault are not reported to the police.

Investigations and management

In this case, there are certain areas that need to be investigated: the domestic physical abuse, the serious sexual assault and the pregnancy itself. Issues to be kept in mind include confidentiality, safeguarding and support of the woman.

The woman is entitled to patient confidentiality, and documentation should be written in a way that would maintain confidentiality. If there are other children in the family, safeguarding issues will arise and referral to social services will be needed. In every case, a multidisciplinary approach is important. Every Trust should have a named midwife/consultant dealing with these cases. The woman should be offered access to a range of services, including reporting the case to the police, access to women's refuge and written info/online resources for help and support.

In cases of sexual assault, issues that need to be addressed include:

- The woman should be assessed by appropriately trained healthcare professionals
- The history of the event should be taken in a sensitive and non-judgemental way
- Assess any injuries sustained after obtaining consent–early evidence kit should be available
- Assess the risk of pregnancy
- Consider emergency contraception: options include copper intrauterine device, Ulipristal acetate orally and 1.5 mg of levonorgestrel orally
- Assess the risk of sexually transmitted infections–screen after 10 to 14 days, but start human immunodeficiency virus postexposure prophylaxis after sexual exposure (PEPSE) within 24 hours if possible or 72 hours maximum, and take for 28 days
- Mental health assessment (especially assessment for posttraumatic stress disorder)

It is useful to know the following in terms of forensic samples' time frame (Table 10.1).

Table 10.1

Forensic Samples' Timeframe[6]	
Type of penetration	**Time frame**
Penile	
Oral penetration	2 days
Vaginal penetration	7 days
Anal penetration	3 days
Digital penetration	2 days
Skin swabs	2 days or 7 days if not washed

KEY POINTS

- Domestic violence is common in the United Kingdom with one in four women having experienced it

- Pregnancy increases the risk of a woman being abused, and domestic abuse increases the risks of pregnancy itself

- UK law clearly defines sexual assault

- Sexual assault is an underreported crime in the United Kingdom

- Women reporting sexual assault should be offered access to various services and be managed by the appropriate team

References

1. Wokoma TT et al; A comparative study of the prevalence of domestic violence in women requesting a termination of pregnancy and those attending the antenatal clinic. *BJOG* 2014 Apr;121(5):627–633.
2. World Health Organization. Violence against women – Intimate partner and sexual violence against women. Fact sheet, 2017. http://www.who.int/mediacentre/factsheets/fs239/en/
3. Long L, Butler B. Sexual assault. London: TOG; 2018.
4. Sexual offences Act 2003: Chapter 42. www.legislation.gov.uk/ukpga/2003/42/contents
5. elearning.rcog.org.uk; core knowledge; domestic abuse and substance misuse
6. elearning.rcog.org.uk; core knowledge; rape and forensic gynaecology

Issues Pertinent to Migrant Women—Female Genital Mutilation

NEKTARIA VAROUXAKI • SHREELATA DATTA

Case

A 25-year-old-woman from Egypt attended her general practitioner (GP) surgery complaining of recurrent urinary tract infections. During history taking, she was noted to complain of superficial dyspareunia as well as painful menstrual periods. She migrated to the United Kingdom with her parents from Egypt at the age of 13 years and is otherwise fit and well. She had never been pregnant. She got married 3 years ago, and this has been the only relationship she has had.

On examination by the GP, a type 3 female genital mutilation (FGM) was noted. The woman reported that the FGM was performed at the age of 9 years in Egypt. The GP discussed in detail with the woman and explained the data recording process, as well as the law that applies to FGM in the United Kingdom. He referred her to the designated gynaecology outpatient clinic, where deinfibulation under local anaesthetic was discussed and arranged. She was also referred for psychologic assessment.

Introduction and epidemiology

FGM is defined as all procedures involving partial or total removal of the external female genitalia or other injury to female genital organs for non-medical reasons. The World Health Organization classifies FGM in Table 11.1.[1]

It is usually carried out in girls between infancy and 15 years of age. Prevalence of FGM varies significantly between different countries, with Somalia and Guinea having the highest rates at 98% and 96%, respectively. Egypt has a prevalence of 91%.[3]

Table 11.1

The World Health Organization Female Genital Mutilation Classification	
Type 1	Partial or total removal of the clitoris and/or prepuce (clitoridectomy)
Type 2	Partial or total removal of the clitoris and the labia minora, with or without excision of the labia majora (excision)
Type 3	Narrowing of the vaginal orifice with creation of a covering seal by cutting and appositioning the labia minora and/or the labia majora, with or without excision of the clitoris (infibulation)
Type 4	All other harmful procedures to the female genitalia for non-medical purposes, such as pricking, piercing, incising, scraping and cauterization

Clinical presentation

A woman might attend because of an acute complication of FGM, such as haemorrhage, urinary retention, genital swelling or fever caused by infection. She might also seek advice because of the long-term complications of FGM. These include genital scarring, urinary tract complications (as the woman in the earlier case), impaired sexual function, psychologic disorders, obstetric complications and complications related to menstrual periods (haematocolpos and dysmenorrhoea).

Investigations

FGM has been a crime in the United Kingdom since 1985. The FGM Act 2003 states that 'FGM is illegal unless it is necessary for the girl's/woman's physical or mental health or is related to labour/birth. It is also illegal to arrange or assist in arranging for any UK resident/national to go overseas for FGM. Reinfibulation is also illegal and should not be performed under any circumstances.'

Any recent FGM or FGM performed on a woman younger than 18 years of age should be reported to the police and/or social services.

Management

Data recording is mandatory for all women with FGM. The type of FGM as well as further details should be documented according to the Health and Social Care Information Centre FGM Enhanced dataset requirements. The data is anonymised after the statistical analysis has been performed, and the woman should be aware of that.[4]

If the woman has attended the designated gynaecology outpatient clinic, she should be assessed for deinfibulation under local anaesthetic, and this should ideally be done before the woman's first intercourse. Referral for psychologic assessment should also be discussed, as well as screening for sexually transmitted diseases and testing for human immunodeficiency virus, hepatitis B and hepatitis C.[2]

If the FGM is diagnosed during pregnancy, the woman should be referred to the designated consultant led clinic. Deinfibulation will be discussed and is preferably performed antenatally at approximately 20 weeks. It can also be done during the first stage of labour, during delivery or even during caesarean section. All women should be asked about FGM during their pregnancy. FGM should be reported whenever an unborn child or other child is at risk. If a baby girl is born from a mother who has undergone FGM, the child protection midwife should be notified and the mother's FGM is documented in the baby's Red book (regardless of baby's sex).[2]

KEY POINTS

- There are four types of female genital mutilation (FGM)
- The countries with the highest prevalence are Somalia and Guinea
- There are short-term and long-term complications of FGM
- FGM is illegal in the United Kingdom
- Women could be seen while pregnant or in an outpatient gynaecology setting because of complications of FGM
- Data recording is compulsory for all women with FGM, whereas reporting to the police and/or social services is only mandatory in certain cases

References

1. World Health Organization. (2008). *Eliminating female genital mutilation: An interagency statement.* Geneva: World Health Organization.
2. RCOG. (2015). Green-Top Guideline No 53, Female genital mutilation and its management.
3. United Nations Children's Fund. Female Genital Mutilation/Cutting. A statistical overview and exploration of the dynamics of change. New York: Unicef;2013.
4. Eealth and Social Care Information Centre. Female Genital Mutilation (FGM) Enhanced Dataset. Requirements Specification {Leeds}: HSIC;2015.

Toxic Shock Syndrome

SAI GNANASAMBANTHAN • SHREELATA DATTA

Case

A 15-year-old girl presented to the emergency department complaining of a headache, hot and cold flashes, abdominal pain and vomiting. She also described a tender rash that started around the perineum and spread to her thighs, legs and hands. On obtaining a thorough history, her last menstrual period was 1 week before her presentation, during which she used tampons. She also disclosed that she changed tampons infrequently, often forgetting to change daily. Her temperature was 37.8°C, with a blood pressure of 99/62 mm Hg, respiration rate of 16 breaths per minute and pulse of 105 beats per minute. Her abdomen was soft, with tenderness in the epigastric area and no peritonism or masses. Her vulva was erythematous, swollen and tender, with no discharge or rash visible. Bloods were taken, including cultures (which only showed a raised white cell count of 13), and she was commenced on intravenous (IV) clindamycin 900 mg, three times a day for 3 days. This was then stepped down to the oral form (300 mg four times a day), as she was apyrexic with improving bloods, for a further 4 days to complete a course of 7 days and was discharged home with advice on avoiding tampon use during periods.

Introduction and epidemiology

Toxic shock syndrome (TSS), although rare, is a life-threatening condition. It is an exotoxin-mediated illness commonly caused by either methicillin-resistant *Staphylococcus aureus* (MRSA) or group A streptococcus (*Streptococcus pyogenes*) bacteria. These bacteria, once within the bloodstream, can release toxins that cause organ damage, septic shock and death if not treated quickly. Risk factors include tampons (particularly high-absorbency tampons) that are left in for longer than recommended (menstrual cause), use of female barrier contraceptives (diaphragm or contraceptive cap), skin breaks including cuts and burns, and nasal packing for nosebleeds (non-menstrual causes). Annual incidence in the United Kingdom is 0.07 per 100,000. Children less than 16 years old accounted for 39% of cases; however, these cases are mostly caused by burns and skin or soft tissue infections. *Staphylococcus* is responsible for 95% of menstrual-related TSS and 50% of non-menstrual TSS. Menstrual and non-menstrual TSS are identical clinically. Some 95% of patients diagnosed with menstrual TSS have onset of illness during menses. Staphylococcal TSS has an associated 5% mortality in menstrual related cases, with non-menstrual TSS having a two to three times higher mortality rate. Recurrence rate is up to 40% in patients who do not generate an appropriate antibody response.[1]

Clinical presentation: signs and symptoms

Symptoms start suddenly and worsen quickly; therefore prompt recognition and appropriate management are crucial. Patients often present with non-specific signs and symptoms like pyrexia and flu-like symptoms (headache, muscle aches and a sore throat). They can also complain of nausea and diarrhoea, and a rash. Local pain or oedema may also occur. Worsening symptoms include syncope, difficulty breathing, confusion and drowsiness. Signs include a raised temperature, tachycardia, raised respiration rate and lowered Glasgow Coma Scale.

Investigations

Initial investigations include microscopy and culture of blood (<5% are positive in staphylococcus TSS), wound, fluid, urine or tissue followed by a full blood count (FBC), clotting investigations, C-reactive protein and renal function. A chest x-ray should be performed as part of the septic screen but should not delay commencing antibiotic treatment.

Management

Once the condition is suspected, prompt management is vital to prevent deterioration of the patient and, worse, death. Once sepsis is identified, treatment with IV antibiotics needs to be started within the 'golden hour'. IV antibiotics need to be broad spectrum and in keeping with local guidelines and the patients' allergy status.

Advice can be obtained from the microbiology team if required. Usual first-line treatment is IV clindamycin 900 mg, three times a day for 3 days, which can then be stepped down to the oral form (300 mg four times a day). IV vancomycin can also be considered if MRSA is suspected. Prompt removal of a retained tampon or barrier contraception should be carried out together with vaginal swabs for microscopy and culture.[2] Vaginal irrigation with betadine solution can be considered. Oxygen should be given to help with breathing, and IV fluids help prevent dehydration and organ damage. If blood pressure and heart rate cannot be controlled quickly, critical care or outreach teams need to be called to assess if the patient needs admission to the intensive care unit for management. In severe cases, dialysis may be required also. Commencing IV immunoglobulin G (IVIG) should be considered if there is no clinical response within the first 6 hours of IV antibiotics. Prevention includes treating wounds quickly and seeking medical advice if there are signs of developing infections, changing tampons regularly, using only one at a time, alternating them with sanitary towels or panty liners and remembering to remove them at the end of the period, all the while practicing good hand hygiene during handling. It is advised that use of tampons or female barrier contraception be avoided if the patient has had toxic shock syndrome before.

KEY POINTS

- TSS is rapidly progressing and fatal if not recognized and treated promptly

- Menstrual-related and non-menstrual-related TSS are commonly caused by staphylococcus and streptococcus bacteria

- Symptoms and signs are non-specific

- Investigations include a general septic screen and removal of the offending product

- Treatment involves broad-spectrum antibiotics within the 'golden hour' and stabilising the patient

References

1. DeVries AS, Lesher L, Schlievert PM, Rogers T, Villaume LG, Danila R, et al. Staphylococcal toxic shock syndrome 2000–2006: epidemiology, clinical features, and molecular characteristics. *PLoS ONE* 2011;6(8):e22997.
2. Lappin E, Ferguson AJ. Gram-positive toxic shock syndromes. *Lancet Infect Dis* 2009;9:281–290.

Cervical Screening in Pregnancy

NEKTARIA VAROUXAKI • SHREELATA DATTA

Case

A 32-year-old woman presented at 29 weeks' gestation in her first pregnancy because of vaginal spotting over the last 2 days. There was no abdominal pain and she experienced regular foetal movements. Placenta was anterior and high on her anomaly scan at 20 weeks. Her smear test results were normal and up to date with the last one done approximately 1 year prior. On speculum examination, there was no active bleeding. However, the cervix appeared abnormal/suspicious. She was referred for colposcopy. The colposcopic impression was of cervical intraepithelial neoplasia (CIN) 1, so a plan was made to repeat the colposcopy 3 months post delivery.

Introduction and epidemiology

Cervical pathology is a key cause of antepartum haemorrhage, which can easily be overlooked. The incidence of cervical cancer during pregnancy is low at 7.5 cases per 100,000 deliveries.[3] Pregnancy itself has no adverse effect on the prognosis. Moreover, pregnant women with borderline nuclear changes or low-grade dyskaryosis rarely have high grade changes at colposcopy that require biopsy during pregnancy. However, cervical screening, as well as follow-up, should be considered separately during pregnancy.

Clinical presentation

There are several different possible scenarios in terms of cervical screening and colposcopy during pregnancy.

A woman might be symptomatic, most commonly complaining of postcoital bleeding/spotting or vaginal discharge, and a cervical lesion might be noted on speculum examination as described in the earlier case. The presentation of cervical cancer in pregnancy depends on the stage at diagnosis and lesion size; most women with International Federation of Gynecology and Obstetrics (FIGO) stage 1 cervical cancer are asymptomatic.[2,3]

Other women might get pregnant during the follow-up period after colposcopy or even treatment for CIN 2/3 or cervical glandular intraepithelial neoplasia (cGIN).

Investigations and management

According to the National Health Service Cervical Screening Programme – Colposcopy and programme management – the investigation and management of women during pregnancy should follow the criteria described here:[1]

- If a woman has been called for routine screening and she is pregnant, the test should be deferred until 3 months after delivery.

- A woman referred with abnormal cytology should undergo colposcopy in late first or early second trimester unless there is a clinical contraindication; however, for low-grade changes triaged to colposcopy on the basis of a positive human papilloma virus (HPV) test, the woman's assessment may be delayed until after delivery.

- If a previous colposcopy was abnormal and in the interim the woman becomes pregnant, colposcopy should not be delayed.

- If a pregnant woman requires colposcopy or cytology after treatment (or follow-up of untreated CIN1), her assessment may be delayed until after delivery. Unless there is an obstetric contraindication, however, assessment should not be delayed if the first appointment for follow-up cytology or colposcopy is due following treatment for cGIN. The 'test of cure' appointment should not be delayed after treatment for CIN2 or CIN3 with involved or uncertain margin status.

- The colposcopist may wish to perform colposcopy only at a follow-up appointment scheduled during pregnancy.

- If repeat cytology is due, and the woman has missed or cancelled her appointment before pregnancy, cytology or colposcopy during pregnancy can be considered.

  - A woman who meets the criteria for colposcopy should be examined in the colposcopy clinic even if she is pregnant. The primary aim of colposcopic examination of a pregnant woman is to exclude invasive disease and to defer biopsy or treatment until the woman has delivered. Women seen in early pregnancy may require a further assessment in the late second trimester at the clinician's discretion.

- If colposcopy has been performed during pregnancy, post-partum assessment of women with an abnormal cytology or biopsy-proven CIN is essential (3 months postpartum). Excision biopsy in pregnancy cannot be considered thera-peutic, and these women should be seen for postpartum colposcopy. A system must be in place to ensure women are given an appointment after delivery.

- Colposcopic evaluation of the pregnant woman requires a high degree of skill:

- If CIN1 or less is suspected, repeat the examination 3 months following delivery.

- If CIN2 or CIN3 is suspected, repeat colposcopy at the end of the second trimester. If the pregnancy has already advanced beyond that point, repeat 3 months following delivery.

- If invasive disease is suspected clinically or colposcopically, a biopsy adequate to make the diagnosis is essential.

KEY POINTS

- The incidence of cervical cancer in pregnancy is low, and pregnancy itself has no adverse effect on the prognosis

- If the cervix appears clinically suspicious or abnormal, the woman should be referred for colposcopy

- The primary aim of colposcopic examination of a pregnant woman is to exclude invasive disease and to defer biopsy or treatment until the woman has delivered

- If invasive disease is suspected clinically or colposcopically, a biopsy adequate to make the diagnosis is essential

References

1. NHS Cervical Screening Programme- Colposcopy and programme management, NHSCSP Publication Number 20, 3rd ed. 2016. Last update 5 February 2020
2. RCOG. Green-top Guideline No 63: Antepartum Haemorrhage. Last accessed 1 March 2020.
3. Norstrom A et al. Carcinoma of the uterine cervix in pregnancy. A study of the in-cidence and treatment in the western region of Sweden 1973 to 1992. *Acta Obstet Gynecol Scand* 1997;76:583–589.

Chicken Pox in Pregnancy

NUALA COYLE • SHREELATA DATTA

Case

A 30-year-old G2P1 (patient is currently pregnant and has had one previous delivery) who had recently moved to the United Kingdom from Thailand presented at 20 weeks' gestation with a widespread pruritic erythematous vesicular rash. She reported recent contact with a child with chicken pox. She was unsure if she had ever had chicken pox. Viral swabs were taken from the lesions and sent for polymerase chain reaction (PCR). Varicella-zoster virus immuno-globulin G (VZV IgG) was requested from booking bloods. Results confirmed the patient was nonimmune and this was a case of primary varicella. Acyclovir treatment was commenced. The patient was informed of the risk of foetal varicella syndrome, and a follow-up with foetal medicine was scheduled for 25 weeks' gestation.

Epidemiology

Chicken pox is caused by the varicella zoster virus, a deoxyribo-nucleic acid (DNA) virus of the Herpes family. Clinical presentation can range from a mild febrile illness with rash to more severe infection with systemic symptoms. The incubation period is 1 to 3 weeks. It is a highly infectious virus and is spread by respiratory droplets or direct contact. The disease is infectious 48 hours before appearance of the rash until the vesicles crust over.

Chicken pox is a common childhood illness. Some 90% of adults in the United Kingdom are seropositive for VZV IgG. Primary infection usually confers lifelong immunity. Varicella infection in pregnancy is rare at 3:1000. Women from tropical and subtropical countries are more likely to be seronegative and therefore suscep-tible to infection.

There is currently no vaccination programme in the United Kingdom. Effective vaccination is available; it is a live attenuated vi-rus which can provide immunity for up to 20 years. The vaccination is given in two doses 4 to 8 weeks apart. Women are advised to avoid pregnancy for 4 weeks after completing the two-dose schedule.

Following primary infection, the virus remains dormant in the dorsal root ganglia and may occur in times of stress or reduced immunity. Shingles can be infectious and cause primary VZV infection in a nonimmune individual. This may occur if the shingles affects an exposed area of the skin, for example in herpes zoster opthalmicus.

Clinical presentation: signs and symptoms

Primary infection with varicella in childhood is usually mild and self-limiting. Primary infection in adults may be more severe and can be associated with complications, such as varicella pneumonia. The classical presentation is of a febrile illness associated with skin rash. The rash begins as erythematous clusters of maculopapules, which then become vesicular. The lesions then crust over, usually at about 5 days.

Severe chicken pox may present with respiratory symptoms, widespread rash with mucosal ulceration, haemorrhagic rash, or neurologic symptoms, such as drowsiness.

Reactivation of the virus causes a vesicular erythematous skin rash in a characteristic dermatomal distribution called (herpes zoster) shingles. Shingles in pregnancy is not associated with viraemia, and so the foetus is not at risk.

Investigations

If chicken pox is suspected in pregnancy, viral swabs should be taken and sent for PCR.

In the case of the pregnant patient who has an uncertain history of immunity, serum should be checked for VZV IgG.

Postexposure prophylaxis

In cases whereby nonimmune patients have had significant exposure to chicken pox, varicella zoster immunoglobulin (VZIG) may be administered to prevent infection. VZIG is effective up to for 10 days after exposure. Women should be treated as potentially infectious for 8 to 28 days if they receive VZIG and 8 to 21 days if they do not receive VZIG.

Management

Symptomatic management of the rash and prevention of secondary skin infection should be applied. If the patient presents within 24 hours of the onset of symptoms, Acyclovir (800 mg five times a day for 7 days) should be commenced if more than 20 weeks' gestation. If less than 20 weeks' gestation, it should be considered.

VZIG has no clinical indication in the treatment of chicken pox once symptomatic and a rash has appeared.

All pregnant patients with severe chicken pox should be admitted to a hospital. Women at risk of respiratory complications include smokers, those who are immunosuppressed or take steroids or those have chronic lung disease.

Women who develop chicken pox should be referred to foetal medicine 5 weeks following infection or at 16 to 20 weeks for assessment.

Complications of chicken pox in pregnancy

Maternal complications include varicella pneumonia, hepatitis and encephalitis. Incidence of varicella pneumonia in pregnancy is reported as 5% to 14%.[1]

Vertical transmission to the foetus can be diagnosed by amniocentesis and PCR. The presence of VZV has a high sensitivity for infection but low specificity for development of foetal varicella syndrome (FVS). A negative amniocentesis has a high negative predictive value for the development of FVS.

Chicken pox in the first trimester is not associated with increased risk of miscarriage. If the woman develops chicken pox before 28 weeks' gestation, there is a risk of FVS.

FVS does not occur at the time of initial infection. It is caused by reactivation of the virus in utero. Reported incidence is 0.55% if the infection was during the first trimester, and 0.91% if before 20 weeks.

It is characterised as development of one or more of the following:

- Skin scarring in a dermatomal distribution
- Eye complications (microphthalmia, chorioretinitis or cataracts)
- Limb hypoplasia
- Neurologic complications
  - microcephaly, cortical atrophy, mental retardation or dysfunction of bladder or bowel sphincters.

Antenatal ultrasound diagnosis is possible in cases of:

- Intrauterine growth restriction
- Limb abnormalities
- Microcephaly
- Soft tissue calcification

Magnetic resonance imaging may also be useful if there are findings on ultrasound.

Neonatal varicella infection

If maternal infection occurs in the last 4 weeks of pregnancy, there is risk of transmission to the neonate; up to 50% of neonates are infected and 23% develop clinical varicella. The route of infection may be transplacental: ascending infection or direct contact with lesions.

A neonatologist should be informed, and elective delivery should be delayed for up to 7 days to allow passive transfer of antibodies. The risk of severe infection in the neonate is highest if they are delivered less than 7 days after the development of the rash or if the mother develops the rash within 7 days of delivery. These high-risk neonates should be managed with VZIG prophylaxis with or without Acyclovir. Breastfeeding is not contraindicated.

KEY POINTS

- Varicella zoster is a DNA virus of the herpes family

- Primary infection in pregnancy before 28 weeks' gestation poses a small risk to the foetus, with less than 1% developing foetal varicella syndrome

- Maternal infection should be managed with treatment of symptoms, Acyclovir (500 mg five times a day) if more than 20 weeks' gestation, and an awareness of increased risk of complications in adults – pneumonia, encephalitis and hepatitis

- Neonates born to mothers who developed chicken pox in the last 4 weeks of pregnancy or up to 7 days after delivery are at high risk of developing infection, with 50% developing chicken pox

- Postexposure prophylaxis with varicella zoster immunoglobulin should be given to nonimmune women if there was significant exposure in the last 10 days

References

Lamont RF, Sobel JD, Carrington D, Mazaki-Tovi S, Kusanovic JP, Vaisbuch E, Romero R. Varicella-zoster virus (chickenpox) infection in pregnancy. IJOG 2011;118: 1155–1162.

Royal College of Obstetrics and Gynaecology Green Top Guideline 13 Chicken Pox in Pregnancy, January 2015.

Vaughan JS, Ambros-Rudolph C, Nelson-Piercy, C. Skin disease in pregnancy. BMJ 2014;348:g3489.

Confidentiality

NEKTARIA VAROUXAKI • SHREELATA DATTA

Case

A 15-year-old girl attends the general practitioner (GP) surgery to discuss contraception. She is in a stable consensual relationship for the past 3 months. After obtaining a thorough clinical history and discussing available options, the GP prescribes the combined oral contraceptive. He also counselled the patient regarding barrier contraception and sexually transmitted infections (STIs). He felt that the patient was able to understand all aspects of the advice. She was not willing to inform her parents despite being encouraged by the doctor to involve them. A few days later the mother of the patient attends the surgery angry, requesting details regarding her daughter's visit and prescription. She is claiming that the GP is promoting sexual intercourse at an early age. The GP explains to the mother that he cannot discuss the details she is asking for because of patient confidentiality. He offers to see the mother along with the daughter if this is something they would both agree to do.

Introduction and epidemiology

This scenario could be challenging at several levels for any doctor. It is well known that effective contraception and avoidance of unintended pregnancies is beneficial to women, their families and the health system.

According to the latest release on conception rates in England and Wales by the Office for National Statistics, the under-18 conception rate in 2016 was 18.9 conceptions per thousand women aged 15 to 17 years.[1]

The estimated pregnancy rate of women aged under 16 years fell by 19% between 2015 and 2016 (2821 in 2016, compared with 3466 in 2015).

In terms of legal abortions, women aged under 16 years had the highest percentage (61.5%).

Therefore it is important to be able to counsel and provide young women with effective advice and treatment.

At the same time, it is of paramount importance to assess if the patient is Gillick competent and to maintain patient confidentiality as you would for an adult patient.

Management

The General Medical Council (GMC) advises the following regarding women under 16 years old:[2]

"You can provide contraceptive, abortion and STI advice and treatment, without parental knowledge or consent, to young people under 16 years provided that:

a. they understand all aspects of the advice and its implications

b. you cannot persuade the young person to tell their parents or to allow you to tell them

c. in relation to contraception and STIs, the young person is very likely to have sex with or without such treatment

d. their physical or mental health is likely to suffer unless they receive such advice or treatment, and

e. it is in the best interests of the young person to receive the advice and treatment without parental knowledge or consent."

The GMC also states the following regarding confidentiality in patients aged less than 18 years:[2]

"Respecting patient confidentiality is an essential part of good care; this applies when the patient is a child or young person as well as when the patient is an adult. Without the trust that confidentiality brings, children and young people might not seek medical care and advice, or they might not tell you all the facts needed to provide good care.

The same duties of confidentiality apply when using, sharing or disclosing information about children and young people as about adults. You should:

a. disclose information that identifies the patient only if this is necessary to achieve the purpose of the disclosure – in all other cases you should anonymise the information before disclosing it

b. inform the patient about the possible uses of their information, including how it could be used to provide their care and for clinical audit

c. ask for the patient's consent before disclosing information that could identify them, if the information is needed for any other purpose, other than in the exceptional circumstances described in this guidance

d. keep disclosures to the minimum necessary."

"*Sharing information with the right people can help to protect children and young people from harm and ensure that they get the help they need. It can also reduce the number of times they are asked the same questions by different professionals. By asking for their consent to share relevant information, you are showing them respect and involving them in decisions about their care.*

If children and young people are able to take part in decision-making, you should explain why you need to share information, and ask for their consent. They will usually be happy for you to talk to their parents and others involved in their care or treatment.

If a child or young person does not agree to disclosure there are still circumstances in which you should disclose information:

a. when there is an overriding public interest in the disclosure

b. when you judge that the disclosure is in the best interests of a child or young person who does not have the maturity or understanding to make a decision about disclosure

c. when disclosure is required by law.

If you judge that disclosure is justified, you should disclose the information promptly to an appropriate person or authority and record your discussions and reasons. If you judge that disclosure is not justified, you should record your reasons for not disclosing.

You must disclose information as required by law. You must also disclose information when directed to do so by a court."

KEY POINTS

- Contraception can be prescribed for women under 16 years old if they are found to be Gillick competent

- Patient confidentiality should be maintained

- Disclosure of information is only allowed if the young person is at risk of neglect, abuse or harm; if it is required by law; or if there is an overriding public interest in the disclosure.

References

1. Ons.gov.uk: conception rates in England and Wales, released in March 2018
2. General Medical Council. GMC ethical guidance for doctors: 0-18 years. 2018. https://www.gmc-uk.org/ethical-guidance/ethical-guidance-for-doctors/0-18-years.

Contact Tracing

NEKTARIA VAROUXAKI • SHREELATA DATTA

Case

A 21-year-old woman attended her general practitioner (GP) office because of increased purulent vaginal discharge for approximately 2 weeks. She has been sexually active since 16 years of age and has had five new sexual partners over the last 6 months. She is on the combined oral contraceptive and has not been using any barrier contraception. There is no past history of sexually transmitted infections (STIs), and she is otherwise fit and well.

On examination by the GP, abdomen was soft and non-tender and vulva appeared healthy. Offensive discharge was noted, so high vaginal and endocervical swabs were taken. The cervix also appeared inflamed. The swabs came back as chlamydia (+)ive, but gonorrhoea (−)ive. The patient was treated with azithromycin and was counselled regarding STI screening, barrier contraception and contact tracing. Her partners over the last 6 months were offered STI screening, which was accepted by all of them. Three out of the five men were chlamydia (+)ive. The method of partner notification for each partner was documented, as well as the partner notification outcomes.

Introduction/epidemiology

Chlamydia trachomatis is an obligate intracellular bacterium which is known to cause genital chlamydial infection. Serotypes D–K cause urogenital infection, whereas L1–L3 cause lymphogranuloma venereum (LGV).

Chlamydia is the most commonly reported curable bacterial STI in the United Kingdom.[3] The highest prevalence rates are noted in 15- to 24-year-olds and are estimated between 1.5% and 10% in different studies (Box 16.1).

Box 16.1 Chlamydia Risk Factors

Age <25 years
New partner over last year
Poor socio-economic status
Use of non-barrier contraception
Infection with other sexually transmitted infection

Box 16.2 Pelvic Inflammatory Disease

Tubal subfertility
Ectopic pregnancy
Fitz-Hugh-Curtis (liver capsule inflammation and adhesions)
Reiter's syndrome: arthritis-conjunctivitis-urethritis

Infection is primarily through penetrative sexual intercourse. If untreated, infection may persist or resolve spontaneously, with up to 50% of infections spontaneously resolving approximately 12 months from initial diagnosis.

Complications of chlamydial infection in women include the following in Box 16.2.

Clinical presentation: signs and symptoms

The majority of chlamydial infections remain asymptomatic. If a woman develops symptoms of the infection, these include increased/offensive per vagina discharge, dysuria, dyspareunia, intermenstrual/postcoital bleed and lower abdominal pain. On examination, mucopurulent discharge can be noted, as well as a red and friable cervix with or without contact bleeding. There might also be pelvic tenderness or cervical motion tenderness. If the male partner is symptomatic, he will be complaining of urethral discharge.

Investigations

The 2015 British Association for Sexual Health and HIV (BASHH) guideline on the management of infection with *Chlamydia trachomatis* advises the following: "Testing for genital and extra-genital chlamydia should be performed using NAATs."[1] Vulvovaginal swab is the specimen of choice for women. This is collected by inserting a dry swab about 2 to 3 inches into the vagina and gently rotating for 10 to 30 seconds. It has a sensitivity of 96% to 98% and has the additional advantage that the sample can be obtained by the woman herself.

Moreover, there is a high rate of co-existence of gonorrhoea, with rates as high as 40%. Therefore, all patients diagnosed with *C. trachomatis* should be encouraged to have screening for other STIs, including HIV, and, where indicated, hepatitis B screening and vaccination. If the patient is within the window periods for HIV and syphilis, these should be repeated at an appropriate time interval.

All patients identified with C. trachomatis should have partner notification discussed at the time of diagnosis by a trained health-care professional. Approximately 60% to 70% of sexual contacts will be chlamydia (+)ive.

All sexual partners should be offered, and encouraged to take up, full STI screening, including HIV testing and, if indicated, hepatitis B screening and vaccination.

Regarding the look-back period, the BASHH guideline advises the following:

- Male index cases with urethral symptoms: all contacts since, and in the four weeks before, the onset of symptoms.

- All other index cases (i.e. all females, asymptomatic males and males with symptoms at other sites, including rectal, throat and eye): all contacts in the six months before presentation.

> *"It is important to remember that repeat testing should be performed 3 to 6 months after treatment only in under 25 year olds diagnosed with chlamydia.*
>
> *The specimen of choice in men for the diagnosis of chlamydial infections is first-catch urine. It is easy to collect, does not cause discomfort and has a high sensitivity. The male patient should be advised to hold his urine for at least 1 hour before collecting the sample and to include the first 20 mL of urine because this contains the highest viral load".*

Management

Recommended regimens for the treatment of uncomplicated genital chlamydial infections are:

- Doxycycline 100 mg twice a day (bd) orally for 7 days
- Ofloxacin 400 mg once daily (OD) for 7 days (alternative regimen)
- Erythromycin 500 mg BD for 10 to 14 days (alternative regimen)

BASHH no longer recommends single-dose azithromycin for treatment of uncomplicated chlamydia infection at any site, regardless of the gender of the infected individual.[2]

Doxycycline 100 mg bd for 7 days is now recommended as first-line treatment for uncomplicated urogenital, pharyngeal and rectal chlamydia infections, with test of cure (TOC) for diagnosed rectal infections (updated 26 September 2018).[2]

Individuals co-infected with gonorrhoea and rectal chlamydia should be treated with ceftriaxone, azithromycin and doxycycline.

Patients should be advised to avoid genital, oral and anal sex until treatment has been completed. After treatment with doxycycline, patients may resume sexual activity at the end of the 7-day course.

TOC is only recommended in pregnancy, where poor compliance is suspected and where symptoms persist.[2]

KEY POINTS

- Infection with *Chlamydia trachomatis* is the most common bacterial sexually transmitted infection in the United Kingdom.

- The majority of cases are diagnosed in individuals aged less than 25 years

- Most patients will be asymptomatic

- Diagnosis is made via nucleic acid amplification tests

- Contact tracing is advised, and sexual intercourse should be avoided until treatment of index patient and partner(s) has been completed

- Some 60% to 70% of sexual contacts will be chlamydia (+)ive

References

1. Nwokolo NC, Dragovic B, Patel S, Tong W, Barker G, Radcliffe K. BASHH 2015 UK national guideline for the management of infection with Chlamydia trachomatis. *Int J STD AIDS* 2016;27:251–267.
2. BASHH update to first line treatment recommendation for uncomplicated chlamydial infection, 26 September 2018.
3. Adams EJ et al. Chlamydia trachomatis in the United Kingdom: a systematic review and analysis of prevalence studies. *Sex Transm Infect*. 2004 Oct;80(5):354–362.

Contraception for Postpartum Women

ANNETTE THWAITES • USHA KUMAR

Case

Joy is a 37-year-old, black Caribbean woman 9 weeks postpartum. She has three children aged 8 years, 6 years and 9 weeks. She attends the sexual health clinic, with her baby, requesting the 'copper coil' which she has used previously in her late 20s and again before her most recent pregnancy. The copper intrauterine device (IUD) has previously suited her well, although she does remember that her periods had been heavy and painful. All her children have been born by caesarean section (for failure to progress, breech and elective reasons), and she feels very sure that her family is now complete. There were several intramural and subserosal fibroids noted on her antenatal ultrasound scans, but she has no other medical history. She has been mixed-feeding (breast and bottle) and has not had a period since delivery.

She has been intending to get her coil fitted for the last 5 weeks, but her baby has had multiple appointments in the tongue-tie clinic, her eldest child was unwell and then it was the school half-term holidays and she had no childcare. She had tried to make an appointment 3 weeks ago but was told there were no appointments available. She did attend the walk-in clinic later that week but was told that the wait for an IUD was over an hour and she left after 45 minutes, as her baby daughter was crying and Joy was having difficulty feeding her in the waiting room. Joy is upset when her pregnancy test is positive today. She was shocked, as she did not think she could get pregnant before her first period and while breastfeeding. She is already finding it difficult recovering from her last delivery and says she is unsure if she would be able to cope with another baby, especially so soon.

You discuss the pregnancy options with Joy. She feels termination and adoption are not right for her and wants to discuss the pregnancy with her husband and sister. You assess Joy for symptoms of postnatal depression and risk of self-harm/harm to her children and are satisfied that there is no evidence of this. You arrange to see her again to discuss her contraceptive needs following this pregnancy. You mention that having a coil fitted at the time of her next delivery is a safe, effective option, and that the Mirena® coil often reduces menstrual bleeding also.

Introduction

In the United Kingdom, one in six pregnancies are unplanned and 45% are unplanned or ambivalent according to the third British National Survey of Sexual Attitudes and Lifestyles (Natsal-3).[1] Postnatal women are at risk of rapid repeat, unplanned pregnancy with associated adverse outcomes for mother and child. Currently, the World Health Organization (WHO) recommends a 24-month interpregnancy interval after childbirth,[2] and an interpregnancy interval of less than 12 months increases the risk of preterm birth, low birth weight, stillbirth and neonatal death.[3]

Recent Faculty of Sexual and Reproductive Healthcare guidance states that maternity service providers should ensure that all women have access to the full range of effective contraceptive methods, including long-acting reversible contraception (LARC), and be able to provide these immediately after childbirth before discharge from the place of delivery.[4] However, this is not currently routine clinical practice across UK National Health Service (NHS) maternity hospitals, and a recent UK study found that almost 1 in 13 women presenting for abortion or delivery had conceived within 1 year of giving birth.[5]

Contraception after childbirth should be initiated by day 21 in order to be effective before ovulation resumes, and if hormonal methods are initiated 21 days or after, additional precautions (barrier/abstinence) are required until the method has become effective. Similarly, emergency contraception is indicated for women who have had unprotected sexual intercourse from 21 days after childbirth. A woman's chosen method of contraception can, however, be safely initiated immediately after childbirth if she is medically eligible. The provision of LARC, immediately postnatally, including intrauterine methods at the time of caesarean section, has also been shown to be safe and effective in preventing rapid repeat pregnancy.

Clinical presentation

The 6-week postnatal general practitioner (GP) check has traditionally been thought of as the opportunity to discuss and address a woman's postnatal contraception needs. However, ovulation can occur as early as 28 days postpartum, and approximately 50% of women have resumed sexual activity before 6 weeks.[6] Moreover, new mothers are faced with multiple barriers to accessing effective and timely contraception in the community. Not all GP practices routinely offer postnatal checks or the full range of the most effective LARC methods, and those that do require more than one appointment. There is evidence of low rates of return for a postnatal contraception visit among postnatal women who have indicated a desire for postnatal intrauterine methods[7] even on 'fast-track' pathways.[8] Providing immediate postnatal contraception at the place of delivery is one way to overcome these barriers and provide a unique opportunity to reach more vulnerable groups, including women with drug, alcohol or mental health problems, who may not attend for routine postnatal care or proactively seek contraception.[9]

It is therefore recommended that all healthcare professionals providing reproductive healthcare should recognise and maximise every opportunity during the antenatal, intrapartum and postnatal periods to provide information and counsel women on the contraceptive choices available to them after birth and be able to provide their chosen methods immediately.[4] Good pathways with specialist contraception services should also be ensured for women with complex conditions or needs.

Contraception

The UKMEC categories for the postpartum period and while breastfeeding are shown in Table 17.1. Health professionals must ensure women are supported antenatally and postnatally to make an informed choice of method of postpartum contraception. When counselling women on postpartum contraception, women should also be informed about the effectiveness of the different contraceptive methods, including the superior effectiveness of LARC,[4] as well as addressing safety concerns. Digital toolkits on contraceptive choices postpregnancy can be helpful when counselling women.[10]

For women with no other medical conditions, all progestogen-only methods, including all LARC (intrauterine methods, implants and injectables), are safe immediately postnatally and when breastfeeding.[11] The progestogen-only pill (POP) and progestogen-only implant are UK medical eligibility criteria (UKMEC) category 1 at all times postnatally, including immediately after delivery, in breastfeeding and nonbreastfeeding women. Because of theoretical concerns that use of depo-medroxyprogesterone acetate (DMPA) may be associated with an increased risk of venous thromboembolism (VTE) compared with other progestogen-only methods, the UKMEC classification is higher for DMPA (UKMEC 2) than the implant and

Table 17.1

UK Medical Eligibility Criteria Summary Table Hormonal and Intrauterine Contraception for Postpartum and Breastfeeding Women[11]						
Condition	**Cu-IUD**	**LNG-IUS**	**IMP**	**DMPA**	**POP**	**CHC**
Personal characteristics and reproductive history						
BREASTFEEDING						
a. 0 to <6 weeks			1	2	1	4
b. ≥6 weeks to <6 months (primarily breastfeeding)		See below	1	1	1	2
c. ≥6 months			1	1	1	1
POSTPARTUM (IN NONBREASTFEEDING WOMEN)						
a. 0 to <3 weeks						
i. With other risk factors for VTE			1	2	1	4
ii. Without other risk factors		See below	1	2	1	3
b. 3 to <6 weeks						
i. With other risk factors for VTE			1	2	1	3
ii. Without other risk factors		See below	1	1	1	2
c. ≥6 weeks			1	1	1	1
POSTPARTUM (IN BREASTFEEDING OR NONBREASTFEEDING WOMEN, INCLUDING POSTCAESAREAN SECTION)						
a. 0 to <48 hours	1	1				
b. 48 hours to <4 weeks	3	3				
c. ≥4 weeks	1	1		See above		
d. Postpartum sepsis	4	4				

CHC, Combined hormonal contraception; *Cu-IUD*, copper intrauterine device; *DMPA*, depo-medroxyprogesterone acetate; *IMP*, progestogen-only implant; *LNG-IUS*, levonorgestrel-releasing intrauterine system; *POP*, progestogen-only pill; *VTE*, venous thromboembolism.
Reproduced under licence from FSRH. Copyright © Faculty of Sexual and Reproductive Healthcare 2006 to 2016.

POP (UKMEC 1) for use by women in the first 6 weeks after childbirth. However, there is currently no evidence of a causal link.

Intrauterine contraception is unrestricted (UKMEC 1) in the first 48 hours after uncomplicated caesarean or vaginal birth. Between 48 hours to less than 4 weeks after delivery it is category

UKMEC 3, that is, the theoretical or proven risks usually outweigh the advantages of using the method, and insertion should usually be delayed until 4 weeks, after which its use is again unrestricted (UKMEC 1). The risk of perforation, with vaginal insertion, is low but is independently increased in women who are breastfeeding (relative risk ratio [RR] 4.9, 95% confidence interval [CI], 3.0–7.8) and in the first 36 weeks postpartum (RR 3.0, CI, 1.5–5.4), according to a recent large European study.[12]

In contrast with progestogen-only and immediate intrauterine contraception, the use of oestrogen-containing contraception is heavily restricted in the postpartum period because of increased risk of venous VTE and concerns regarding the effect on breast-feeding. Combined hormonal contraception is largely contraindicated (UKMEC 4 or 3) in first 3 weeks postpartum and UKMEC 3 or 2 in weeks 3 to 6 postpartum, depending on the presence of other VTE risk factors. It is unrestricted after 6 weeks if not breast-feeding. However, if breastfeeding, combined hormonal contraception (CHC) remains a UKMEC 4 for the first 6 weeks and UKMEC 2 between 6 weeks and 6 months postpartum. After 6 months it is unrestricted, that is, UKMEC 1.

All postpartum women must therefore undergo a risk assessment for VTE before prescribing contraception. This should identify risk factors, such as immobility, transfusion at delivery, body mass index (BMI) $\geq$30 kg/m^2, postpartum haemorrhage, caesarean delivery, preeclampsia or smoking. Clinicians should also discuss with women any other medical conditions which may affect her medical eligibility, including any that may have developed in pregnancy. These include gestational hypertension and obstetric cholestasis, which are categorised UKMEC 2 for combined hormonal contraception because of risk of myocardial infarction and VTE and risk of developing combined oral contraceptive-associated cholestasis, respectively.

Immediate postpartum contraception

Women should be advised that most methods can be safely initiated immediately, with the exception of combined hormonal contraception. LARC methods, intrauterine contraception and progestogen-only implant (IMP), can be inserted immediately after delivery and have been shown to be convenient, highly acceptable to women and associated with high continuation rates and a reduced risk of unintended pregnancy.[13] It is to be noted that immediate implant insertion is still currently outside the product licence and that immediate intrauterine contraception is currently still in its infancy in the United Kingdom. Insertion of intrauterine methods, both at vaginal delivery and caesarean section, has been widely used globally with good safety data. There is no increased risk of infection; potentially decreased perforation risk compared with delayed insertion; and, despite higher expulsion rates, higher continuation rates at 6 to 12 months postpartum. Expulsion rates may be lower for insertion at caesarean section compared with immediate insertion post vaginal delivery. Therefore women should be appropriately counselled and given access to prompt replacement.[4]

Effect of contraception on breastfeeding

Women who are breastfeeding should be informed that the available evidence, including multiple systematic reviews,[14,15] indicates that progestogen-only methods of contraception (including levonorgestrel oral emergency contraception (LNG EC)) have no adverse effects on breastfeeding duration, breast milk composition and infant growth or development. A 3-monthly progesterone-releasing vaginal ring, Progering®, specifically designed for breastfeeding women in the first postpartum year to prolong lactational amenorrhea and prevent resumption of ovulation, is available in some Latin American countries. Ulipristal Acetate (UPA) oral emergency contraception is excreted in breast milk, and the effect of this in infants has not been studied, and therefore women should be advised to express and discard breast milk for 1 week after use of UPA. There is currently limited and conflicting evidence regarding the effects of CHC use on breastfeeding and infant outcomes. Women who are breastfeeding should therefore be advised to wait until 6 weeks after childbirth before initiating a CHC method and is categorized as UKMEC 4 before this.

Lactational amenorrhoea method

Breastfeeding itself can be used as a contraceptive method, as suckling suppresses resumption of ovarian activity and the return of menses postpartum. This is known as the lactational amenorrhoea method (LAM). However, this method is associated with strict criteria, which women must be made aware of,[16] and can be a source of confusion.[9]

LAM is over 98% effective at preventing pregnancy only if women are:

- less than 6 months postpartum
- amenorrhoeic (no bleeding after 56 days postpartum) and
- fully breastfeeding

Fully breastfeeding should be further qualified as:

- no other liquids given or only water, juice or vitamins given infrequently in addition to breastfeeds and
- no long intervals between feeds day or night (e.g., >4 hours during day and >6 hours at night)

Women using LAM should therefore be advised that if the frequency of breastfeeding decreases, then ovarian activity may be resumed and the risk of pregnancy is increased. This can occur with the use of dummies/pacifiers, decreased or stopped night feeds and started or increased supplementary feeding with formula or weaning. In addition, the effect of expressing breast milk on the efficacy of LAM is not known but it may potentially be reduced.

Table 17.2 summarises the specific benefits and risks associated with different methods for women in the postpartum period and when breastfeeding.

Table 17.2

Benefits and Risks of Contraceptive Methods		
Type	**Benefits**	**Risks/disadvantages/ considerations**
Cu-intrauterine device (Cu-IUD)	• Highly effective for 5 or 10 years • Can be inserted at the time of caesarean-section or vaginal delivery	• Increased risk of perforation in first 4–36 weeks postpartum ($\times$3) • Increased risk of perforation during vaginal insertion when breast feeding ($\times$5) • Emergency Cu-IUD UKMEC 3 between 3 and 4 weeks postpartum • Practical difficulties associated with women bringing young babies to coil fitting appointments
Intrauterine systems (IUS)	• Highly effective for 3 or 5 years • Can be inserted at the time of caesarean-section or vaginal delivery • May reduce bleeding in puerperium	• Increased risk of perforation in first 4–36 weeks postpartum ($\times$3) • Increased risk of perforation during vaginal insertion when breast feeding ($\times$5) • Practical difficulties associated with women bringing young babies to coil fitting appointments

Continued

Table 17.2

Benefits and Risks of Contraceptive Methods—cont'd		
Type	**Benefits**	**Risks/disadvantages/ considerations**
Nexplanon® implant	• Highly effective for 3 years • Irregular early bleeding may be masked in puerperium • UKMEC 1 at all times postnatally	
Depo-Medroxyprogesterone Acetate (DMPA) injections	• Highly effective • UKMEC 1 or 2 at all times postnatally	• Women should be made aware of potential for problematic bleeding in puerperium
Progestogen only pill (POP)	• UKMEC 1 at all times postnatally	• Medium effectiveness as user dependent
Combined hormonal contraception (CHC)		• Contraindicated (UKMEC 4) in first 6 weeks postpartum if breastfeeding • In nonbreastfeeding women, contraindicated <3 weeks postpartum and UKMEC 3 in weeks 3–6 postpartum if other venous thromboembolism risk factors • Medium effectiveness as user dependent
Emergency oral contraception	• Safe to use postpartum (NB not required before 21 days postpartum) • LNG EC has No known adverse effects on breastfeeding or on breastfed infants	• Effect of UPA on breastfed infants has not been studied. Women should be advised not to breastfeed and to express and discard milk for 1 week after they have taken UPA-EC
Barrier methods	• Condoms provide protection against sexually transmitted infections	• Low effectiveness with higher typical-use failure rates • Diaphragm may no longer fit, and sizing needs to be checked 6 weeks after childbirth before restarting this method

Table 17.2

Benefits and Risks of Contraceptive Methods—cont'd		
Type	Benefits	Risks/disadvantages/ considerations
Laparoscopic sterilisation	• Permanent method	• Increased risk of regret if tubal occlusion performed at the time of delivery • Less effective than some LARC methods • No noncontraceptive benefits

Lactational amenorrhoea method (LAM)	• 98% effective if all criteria met	• women must be:
		  • <6 months postpartum
		  • amenorrhoeic
		  • fully breastfeeding

Fertility awareness methods		• Accurate detection of signs/symptoms of return to fertility and ovulation is unlikely in first 4 weeks after childbirth and in first 6 months postpartum if primarily breastfeeding

KEY POINTS

• Women should be advised that an interpregnancy interval of less than 12 months is associated with an increased risk of preterm birth, low birth weight, stillbirth and neonatal death

• Ovulation can occur as early as 28 days postpartum

• To avoid rapid unplanned pregnancy, women should be advised to use effective contraception from day 21 postpartum

• Health professionals must ensure women are supported antenatally and postnatally to make an informed choice of method of postpartum contraception

• All progestogen-only methods, including long-acting reversible contraception, can be safely initiated immediately after childbirth in breastfeeding and nonbreastfeeding women

• Combined hormonal contraception should not be used in the first 6 weeks postpartum by breastfeeding women but may be considered from 3 weeks postpartum in nonbreastfeeding women with no other risk factors for venous thromboembolism.

- All pregnant and postpartum women should be advised that the lactational amenorrhoea method is only effective if they are less than 6 months postpartum, amenorrhoeic and fully breastfeeding

References

1. Wellings K, Jones KG, Mercer CH, Tanton C, Clifton S, Datta J, et al. The prevalence of unplanned pregnancy and associated factors in Britain: findings from the third National Survey of Sexual Attitudes and Lifestyles (Natsal-3). Lancet 2013;382:1807–1816.
2. World Health Organization. Report of a WHO technical consultation on birth spacing. Geneva: World Health Organization; 2006.
3. Smith GCS, Pell JP, Dobbie R. Interpregnancy interval and risk of preterm birth and neonatal death: retrospective cohort study. BMJ 2003;327:313.
4. Faculty of Sexual & Reproductive Healthcare. Contraception after pregnancy. 2017. https://www.fsrh.org/standards-and-guidance/documents/contraception-after-pregnancy-guideline-january-2017/. (Accessed 5 March 2021).
5. Heller R, Cameron S, Briggs R, Forson N, Glasier A. Postpartum contraception: a missed opportunity to prevent unintended pregnancy and short inter-pregnancy intervals. J Fam Plann Reprod Health Care 2016;42:93–98.
6. McDonald EA, Brown SJ. Does method of birth make a difference to when women resume sex after childbirth? BJOG 2013;120(7):823–830.
7. Ogburn JA, Espey E, Stonehocker J. Barriers to intrauterine device insertion in postpartum women. Contraception 2005;72(6):426–429.
8. Cameron ST, Craig A, Sim J, Gallimore A, Cowan S, Dundas K, et al. Feasibility and acceptability of introducing routine antenatal contraceptive counselling and provision of contraception after delivery: the APPLES pilot evaluation. BJOG 2017;124:2009–2015.
9. Thwaites A, et al. BMJ Sex Reprod Health 2018;0:1–7. doi:10.1136/bmjsrh-2018-200078
10. CONTRACEPTIVE CHOICES POST-PREGNANCY. The family planning Association. https://www.fpa.org.uk/digital-toolkits-and-webinars/contraceptive-choices-post-pregnancy. (Accessed 5 March 2021).
11. Faculty of Sexual & Reproductive Healthcare. UK medical eligibility criteria for contraceptive Use 2016. 2016. https://www.fsrh.org/standards-and-guidance/external/ukmec-2016-digital- version/ (Accessed 5 March 2021).
12. Barnett C, Moehner S, Do Minh T, Heinemann K. Perforation risk and intra-uterine devices: results of the EURAS-IUD 5-year extension study. Eur J Contracept Reprod Health Care 2017;22(6):424–428.
13. Goldthwaite LM, Shaw KA. Immediate postpartum provision of long-acting reversible contraception. Curr Opin Obstet Gynecol 2015;27:460–464.
14. Lopez LM, Grey TW, Stuebe AM, Chen M, Truitt ST, Gallo MF. Combined hormonal versus nonhormonal versus progestin-only contraception in lactation. Cochrane Database Syst Rev 2015;3:CD003988.
15. Phillips SJ, Tepper NK, Kapp N, Nanda K, Temmerman M, Curtis KM. Progestogen-only contraceptive use among breastfeeding women: a systematic review. Contraception 2016;94:226–252.
16. Faculty of Sexual & Reproductive Healthcare. Fertility awareness methods. 2015. https://www.fsrh.org/standards-and-guidance/documents/ceuguidancefertility-awarenessmethods/ (Accessed 5 March 2021).

Contraception for Women Aged Over 40 Years and in the Perimenopause

ANNA GRAHAM • USHA KUMAR

Case

Paula is 47 years old and attends the clinic for advice regarding contraception, as she has recently embarked upon a new sexual relationship. Her menstrual cycles have changed over the past year with periods becoming infrequent, with cycles ranging from 1 to 3 months. On further questioning, she reveals that she has been experiencing some hot flashes and night sweats. Paula's body mass index (BMI) is 24 kg/m², her blood pressure (BP) is 130/84 mm Hg and she is a non-smoker. Paula wants to know if she still requires contraception and which method would be the best for her.

You advise Paula that she still requires contraception until age 55 years, although her fertility is probably low. You inform her that no contraceptive method is contraindicated on age alone, but there are some that are likely to be more appropriate than others. You explore Paula's thoughts on hormone replacement therapy (HRT), and as you delve further, you also discover that her menopausal symptoms have become quite troublesome, with a low libido, vaginal dryness and superficial dyspareunia. In light of this, you suggest that oestrogen replacement may be something that she could consider, either in the form of combined hormonal contraception (CHC) (no contraindications identified) until age 50 years or a Mirena® intrauterine system (IUS) and additional oestrogen replacement. Paula opts for a Mirena® IUS, and you explain that this can be used for contraception until age 55 years when she no longer requires contraception or if she uses it for endometrial protection in an HRT regimen, then for 5 years. You perform a sexually transmitted infection screen in light of the new partner and insert the Mirena® IUS for Paula.

Introduction and epidemiology

The menopause occurs when a woman reaches the end of her natural reproductive life and the ovaries stop maturing eggs and producing oestrogen and progesterone. It is defined as having occurred when a woman has not had a menstrual period for 12 consecutive months.[1] The average age of the menopause in the United Kingdom is 51 years.[1] The perimenopause is the time leading up to the menopause when a woman experiences irregular cycles of ovulation, typically starting in the mid- to late 40s and lasting 4 to 5 years.[2] During the perimenopause, in response to fluctuating levels of oestrogen, progesterone and follicle-stimulating hormone (FSH), in addition to irregular menstrual bleeding, menopausal symptoms are likely to occur, including vasomotor symptoms, such as hot flashes and night sweats, mood changes, including anxiety and depression, joint and muscle pain, vulvovaginal atrophy and sexual problems.[1,2]

In addition to perimenopausal symptoms, women also have an increased risk of medical issues as they become older, including cardiovascular disease,[3] hypertension, increased risk of venous thromboembolism (VTE) (1:10,000 <40s to 1:1000 aged 40–60 years),[4] osteoporosis,[1] obesity and breast and gynaecological cancers.[5,6]

Data from Public Health England (PHE)[7] also indicates an increase in sexually transmitted diseases in this population as women embark upon internet dating and new sexual relationships.[8]

A woman's fertility declines steeply from age 35 years, with pregnancy rates dropping from approximately 80% for women under 40 years having unprotected sexual intercourse for 1 year, to around 10% to 20% for women aged 40 to 44 years to 12% for women aged 45 to 49 years.[9,10] There has been a significant increase in women over 40 years having babies, which reflects improved assisted conception techniques and women waiting longer because of careers and meeting the right partner[11]; however, older maternal age carries increased risks for mother and baby, including increased caesarean section rates, gestational diabetes and high BP.[2] There is also a significant rise in congenital abnormalities, with the rates of Down Syndrome being 1:1544 at age 20 years but increasing to 1:28 at age 45 years.[12] Particularly striking are the abortion figures in the over 40 years age group, with abortion rates versus live birth rate the highest of all age groups.[13] This data indicate the huge number of unplanned pregnancies within this age group and highlights the essential need for contraception counselling and provision.

Healthcare professionals (HCPs) face significant challenges when prescribing contraception to this age group because of the issues highlighted earlier. This chapter will aim to address the practicalities and challenges faced by HCPs providing contraception in the perimenopause. HRT is beyond the scope of this chapter and will only be addressed in relation to contraception.

Clinical presentation: signs and symptoms

Women can present with a vast array of menopausal symptoms, including vasomotor symptoms such as hot flashes and night sweats, mood changes including anxiety and depression, joint and muscle pain, symptoms of vulvovaginal atrophy such as vaginal dryness, superficial dyspareunia and sexual problems, including reduced libido; additionally, they may just attend requesting contraception or for a sexually transmitted infection screen. Women may not volunteer the symptoms that they are experiencing secondary to embarrassment or not realising they are related to the perimenopause, and therefore it is essential that HCPs ask specific questions particularly around sexual function.[1]

Investigations

The perimenopause and menopause are clinical diagnoses, and it is rarely necessary to perform a hormonal profile. All sexually active women in the perimenopause can be assumed to require contraception. If no contraception or HRT are being used and the woman has not experienced a menstrual period for 1 year, then she can be assumed to be menopausal.[1,2]

A hormone profile to assess menopausal status can be useful in suspected premature ovarian insufficiency (under the age of 40 years) and in women over the age of 50 years who are using hormonal contraception and wish to stop as menopause is suspected. Women over 50 years using progestogen-only contraception (including depo-medroxyprogesterone acetate [DMPA]) can have their FSH levels measured without stopping this method.[2] An FSH over 30 IU/L indicates a degree of ovarian insufficiency but not sterility, and it is recommended that contraception is continued for 1 year after this result.[2] If the woman is using a combined hormonal method of contraception (CHC) or HRT, then the results will not be accurate because of the suppression of FSH, and if necessary to measure, then the CHC or HRT should be stopped for 6 weeks before testing.[2]

Management

Contraception

All contraception methods are available to women between 40 and 49 years of age, assuming eligibility, and women should be assessed for exclusion criteria in the same way that younger women are by referring to the Faculty of Sexual and Reproductive Healthcare UKMEC.[14] No method is contraindicated by age alone until 50 years when CHC should be discontinued and switched to a non-injectable progestogen-only contraception or a non-hormonal method, as the risks of CHC outweigh the benefits. Similarly DMPA users should also be counselled to switch to alternative safer methods after the age of 50 years. When a woman reaches 55 years of age, even if she is still experiencing menstrual bleeding, she can stop all methods of contraception.[2]

Table 18.1 highlights the benefits and risks associated with each method.[2]

Contraception and hormone replacement therapy

HRT will not provide contraceptive cover, and therefore contraception is required. The only contraception that is also licensed for endometrial protection as part of a HRT regimen is the Mirena® IUS, and therefore this should be first-line treatment in combination

Table 18.1

Benefits and Risks of Each Contraceptive Method		
Type	**Benefits**	**Risks and disadvantages**
Combined hormonal contraception (CHC)	• Contraception • Treats menopausal symptoms • Therapeutic option for heavy and irregular menstrual bleeding • Protection against osteoporosis, endometrial cancer and ovarian cancer	• Stop at age 50 years • Increased risk of breast cancer • Increased risk of venous thromboembolism (reduce the risk with CHC containing low dose (≤30 mcg) Ethinyl estradiol and second-generation progestogen, such as Levonorgestrel or Norethisterone)

Table 18.1

Benefits and Risks of Each Contraceptive Method—cont'd		
Type	**Benefits**	**Risks and disadvantages**
Depo-Medroxy-progesterone Acetate (DMPA—Depo-Provera® or Sayana® Press)	• Contraception • Therapeutic option for heavy menstrual bleeding • Protective effect on ovarian and endo-metrial cancers	• Stop at age 50 years • Reduction in bone mineral density (BMD), but initial loss in BMD because of hypoestrogenic effects of DMPA is not repeated or worsened by menopause[15,16] • Weak and conflicting evidence of breast cancer and cardiovascular disease risk
Intrauterine system (IUS): 52 mg Levonorgestrel (LNG)-IUS Mirena®	• Contraception for 10 years if inserted at or after age 45 years[2] • Endometrial protection as part of HRT regimen for 5 years (manufacturer's license for endometrial protection is 4 years, but FSRH supports off-license use for up to 5 years).[2] • Reduction in menstrual blood loss and dysmenorrhoea. • Protection against endometrial cancer • No upper age limit	• Weak and conflicting evidence regarding breast cancer risk • Increased risk of perforation if endometrial ablation has been previously performed • Should not be left in indefinitely because of risk of infection
Intrauterine System (IUS): 52 mg LNG-IUS Levosert® / 19.5 mg LNG-IUS Kyleena® / 13.5 mg LNG-IUS Jaydess®	• Contraception for 6 years with Levosert®, 5 years with Kyleena® and 3 years with Jaydess® • Levosert licensed for treatment of heavy menstrual bleeding • No upper age limit	• Weak and conflicting evidence regarding breast cancer risk • Increased risk of perforation if endometrial ablation has been previously performed • Should not be left in indefinitely because of risk of infection

Continued

Table 18.1

Benefits and Risks of Each Contraceptive Method—cont'd		
Type	**Benefits**	**Risks and disadvantages**
Intrauterine device— copper IUD	• Contraceptive cover 5 or 10 years; can be used for an extended period until menopause if inserted at age 40 years or over A Cu-IUD containing ≥300 mm^2 copper inserted at or after age 40 years can remain in situ until 1 year after the last menstrual period (LMP) if it occurs when the woman is 50 years or older. If a woman is under 50 years, the Cu-IUD can remain in situ for 2 years after the LMP[17]	• May exacerbate heavy menstrual bleeding seen in the perimenopausal period • Should not be left in indefinitely because of risk of infection
Progestogen-only pill (POP)	• Contraceptive cover • No upper age limit	• May exacerbate irregular bleeding
Progestogen only implant - Nexplanon®	• Contraceptive cover for 3 years • No upper age limit • May alleviate menstrual and ovulatory pain • No effect on BMD	• May exacerbate irregular bleeding

with a transdermal oestrogen.[2] If this is not suitable or not acceptable to the woman, then the progestogen-only pill (POP)/DMPA or Nexplanon® can be safely used for contraception in combination with a sequential HRT regimen. At the present time, POP, progestogen-only implant and DMPA are not licensed for and cannot be recommended as endometrial protection with oestrogen-only HRT.[2] CHC can be used in eligible women under 50 years as an alternative to HRT for relief of menopausal symptoms and prevention of loss of bone mineral density.[2] CHC must not be used in combination with HRT.

Use of continuous combined HRT regimens is normally confined to postmenopausal women who, by definition, do not have a requirement for contraception.[2]

KEY POINTS

- Women over 40 years and in the perimenopause require contraception

- They are a challenging group to prescribe for because of increased background medical risks, menstrual problems and perimenopausal symptoms

- No contraception is contraindicated on age alone under 50 years of age

- The Mirena® IUS is licensed for both contraception and endometrial protection during estrogen replacement therapy

- If inserted after age 45 years, then the Mirena® IUS can be used for contraception until age 55 years or the menopause

References

1. National Institute for Health and Care Excellence. Menopause: full guideline. 2015. http://www.nice.org.uk/guidance/ng23/evidence/full-guidance-559549261. (Accessed 5 March 2021).
2. Faculty of Sexual and Reproductive Healthcare. Contraception for women aged over 40 years. 2017. http://www.fsrh.org/standards-and-guidance/documents/cec-ceu-guidance-womenover40-Nov2017. (Accessed 5 March 2021).
3. Hoyt LT, Falconi AM. Puberty and perimenopause: reproductive transitions and their implications for women's health. Soc Sci Med 2015;132:103–112.
4. Scottish Intercollegiate Guidelines Network. Prevention and management of venous thromboembolism. 2014. https://www.sign.ac.uk/media/1060/sign122.pdf (Accessed 5 March 2021).
5. Cancer Research UK. Breast cancer (C50): 2012-2014. http://www.cancerresearchuk.org/sites/default/files/cstream-node/cases_crude_f_breast_I14.pdf. (Accessed 5 March 2021).
6. Cancer Research UK. Ovarian cancer (C56-C57.4): 2012-2014. http://www.cancerresearchuk.org/sites/default/files/cstream-node/cases_crude_ovary_I14.pdf. (Accessed 5 March 2021).
7. Public Health England. Sexually transmitted infections (STIs): annual data tables. Table 2: New STI diagnoses and rates by gender, sexual risk and age group, 2012 to 2016. 2017. http://www.gov.uk/government/statistics/sexually-transmitted-infections-stis-annual-data-tables. (Accessed 5 March 2021).
8. Mercer CH, Tanton C, Prah P, Erens B, Sonnenberg P, Clifton S, et al. Changes in sexual attitudes and lifestyles in Britain through the life course and over time:

findings from the National Surveys of Sexual Attitudes and Lifestyles (Natsal). Lancet 2013;382:1781–1794.

9. Baldwin MK, Jensen JT. Contraception during the perimenopause. Maturitas 2013; 76:235–242.

10. Klein J, Sauer MV. Assessing fertility in women of advanced reproductive age. Am J Obstet Gynecol 2001;185:758–770.

11. Office for National Statistics. Birth summary tables, England and Wales: 2015. 2016. https://www.ons.gov.uk/peoplepopulationandcommunity/birthsdeathsandmarriages/livebirths/datasets/birthsummarytables (Accessed 5 March 2021).

12. Morris JK, Mutton DE, Alberman E. Revised estimates of the maternal age specific live birth prevalence of Down's syndrome. J Med Screen 2002;9:2–6.

13. Office for National Statistics. Conception statistics, England and Wales: 2015. 2017. https://www.ons.gov.uk/peoplepopulationandcommunity/birthsdeathsandmarriages/conceptionandfertilityrates/datasets/conceptionstatisticsenglandandwalesreferencetables (Accessed 5 March 2021).

14. Faculty of Sexual and Reproductive Healthcare. UK medical eligibility criteria 2016. 2016. https://www.fsrh.org/standards-and-guidance/external/ukmec-2016-digital-version/. (Accessed 5 March 2021).

15. Cundy T, Cornish J, Roberts H, Reid IR. Menopausal bone loss in long-term users of depot medroxyprogesterone acetate contraception. Am J Obstet Gynecol 2002;186:978–983.

16. Viola AS, Castro S, Bahamondes MV, Fernandes A, Viola CF, Bahamondes L. A cross-sectional study of the forearm bone mineral density in long-term current users of the injectable contraceptive depot medroxyprogesterone acetate. Contraception 2011;84:e31–e37.

17. Faculty of Sexual & Reproductive Healthcare. Intrauterine contraception. 2015. http://www.fsrh.org/standards-and-guidance/documents/ceuguidanceintrauterinecontraception/. (Accessed 5 March 2021).

Polycystic Ovary Syndrome and Contraception

ANNA GRAHAM • USHA KUMAR

Case

Sarah is 25 years old and has polycystic ovary syndrome (PCOS). She has irregular periods; her last menstrual period was 6 months ago. Her body mass index (BMI) is 36 kg/m^2. Her blood pressure (BP) is 130/88 mm Hg. She has troublesome acne, thinning of her hair, and hirsutism. She is sexually active and does not use any contraception, as she believes that because she has PCOS she cannot fall pregnant. She is not planning a pregnancy in the near future.

Management

Sarah should be counselled about PCOS, including the long-term sequelae, and the need for contraception. She should be given advice about weight loss and exercise to improve her symptoms and prognosis. A urine pregnancy test should be performed three weeks after her last unprotected sexual intercourse to rule out a pregnancy. She has not had a menstrual period for more than 3 months, and therefore after excluding a pregnancy, a withdrawal bleed should be induced, followed by a transvaginal ultrasound scan (TVUSS) to check the endometrial thickness and morphology; if normal, then protection against endometrial hyperplasia and cancer is required, along with contraceptive cover. Combined hormonal contraception is contraindicated because of her high BMI. All progestogen-only methods would be suitable, but the Depo-MedroxyProgesterone Acetate (DMPA) injection could cause increased weight gain. If Sarah were able to lose weight (BMI <35 kg/m^2), then combined hormonal contraception (CHC) could be considered. The safest to use would be one containing a low-dose oestrogen with second-generation progestogen such as Norethisterone or Levonorgestrel.

Introduction and epidemiology

PCOS is a common and complex gynaecological endocrine disorder, including ovulatory dysfunction (oligo/amenorrhoea) and hyperandrogenism leading to hirsutism, alopecia and acne. There are associations with metabolic syndrome, type 2 diabetes, reproductive difficulties, long-term cardiovascular issues and endometrial cancer, secondary to unopposed oestrogen.[1]

The general prevalence is 6%[2–4]; however, 25% of women will have evidence of polycystic ovaries on ultrasound scan but no other symptoms; this is a normal variant and does not require any further investigation.[2–4] Approximately 40% to 50% of patients with PCOS will be overweight (BMI >25 kg/m^2)[4], and a large majority will have a family history of PCOS.[2]

PCOS is named secondary to the appearance of the ovaries on ultrasound scan; however, the 'cysts' described are normal ovarian follicles arrested in an immature state rather than physiologic or pathologic cysts (see Figs.19.1 and 19.2).

The cause of PCOS is currently unknown, but is likely to be multifactorial with both genetic and environmental causes.[4,5] There are a number of theories that currently exist, including:

- Intrinsic ovarian dysfunction
- Hyperinsulinaemia and insulin resistance
- Luteinising hormone hyperstimulation

Intrinsic ovarian dysfunction

Theca cells in PCOS produce increased androgens in response to similar levels of luteinising hormone (LH) compared with normal theca cells.[5,6]

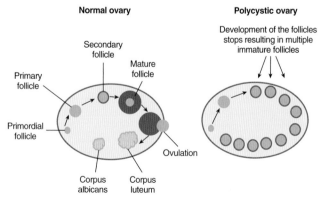

Figure 19.1 A normal ovary versus a polycystic ovary.

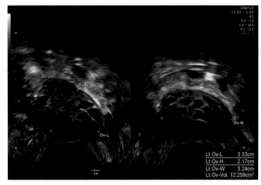

Figure 19.2 Transvaginal ultrasound image of a polycystic ovary.

Hyperinsulinaemia and insulin resistance

Insulin resistance is present in 65% to 80% of women with PCOS independent of obesity.[2] Insulin works with LH to increase androgen production in theca cells and the adrenal gland, leading to saturation of the pathway converting androgens to oestradiol.[5–7] This leads to increased androgen output from the ovaries. Insulin also inhibits the production of sex hormone binding globulin (SHBG), resulting in increased unbound active androgens. It also inhibits insulin-like growth factor 1 binding protein, resulting in further stimulation of theca cells.[4–6]

Luteinising hormone hyperstimulation

LH is elevated in approximately 40% of people with PCOS. It is hypothesised that there is an increased LH pulse frequency and amplitude, resulting in increased androgen production.[5,8]

Clinical presentation: signs and symptoms

Patients present with oligo/amenorrhoea, infertility or clinical signs of hyperandrogenism. The 2003 Rotterdam Consensus on Diagnostic Criteria for PCOS[9] states that two out of the following three need to be present:

- Oligoanovulation (>35-day cycles) or anovulation (>6-month cycles)

- Clinical and/or biochemical signs of hyperandrogenism (raised androgens or hirsutism, acne or alopecia)
- Polycystic ovaries: the presence of 12 or more follicles (measuring 2–9 mm in diameter) in one or both ovaries and/or increased ovarian volume (>10 mL) on ultrasound scan.

However, more recent guidelines have stated that the threshold for polycystic ovarian morphology using transvaginal ultrasound should be ≥ 20 follicles per ovary in either ovary and/or an ovarian volume ≥ 10 ml , and ultrasound should not be used as a diagnostic criteria in women < 8 years after menarche.[10]

Investigations

Table 19.1 lists possible investigations.

A pelvic ultrasound scan can be requested (in adults more than 8 years post-menarche) if the diagnosis is not obvious on clinical and/or biochemical grounds.[10]

Management

Conservative management

Patients require evidence-based advice regarding PCOS, including:

- prevention of and screening for associated long term sequelae, specifically endometrial hyperplasia and type II diabetes
- Weight loss advice if overweight
- Effect on fertility due to absent/infrequent ovulation and
- Need for contraception if not planning a pregnancy, due to unpredictable ovulation
- Screening for depression and anxiety, sexual dysfunction, negative body image and eating disorders[9]

Hormonal treatment

Endometrial protection

If the patient has not had a menstrual bleed in more than 3 months, then a withdrawal bleed should be induced using 10 mg Medroxyprogesterone acetate or 5 mg TDS Norethisterone orally for 14 days. Norethisterone should be used with caution, as it is converted into ethinyl oestradiol and therefore may increase the risk of

Table 19.1

Investigations		
Blood Test	**Normal Range**	**Levels in Polycystic Ovary Syndrome (PCOS)**
For PCOS		
Total testosterone (nmol/L)	0.7–2.6	Normal or high
Sex hormone binding globulin (nmol/L)	40–140	Normal or low
Free androgen index	< 5.0	Normal or high

thromboembolic events.[11] Following this, a TVUSS should be performed to check endometrial thickness and morphology; if more than 10 mm or abnormal in appearance, (see Fig. 19.3) then an endometrial biopsy is required to exclude pathology. If the endometrium is less than 10 mm and appears normal, then ongoing endometrial protection against endometrial hyperplasia and cancer is required.[4] If there is a history of abnormal uterine bleeding, then an urgent TVUSS ± endometrial biopsy should be performed.

Ongoing endometrial protection

There are three suitable options for ongoing endometrial protection which will depend on the patient's individual circumstances:

1. Cyclical progestogen every 3 months. This regime will not provide contraceptive cover and is therefore only suitable for

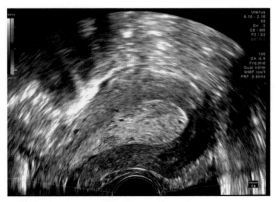

Figure 19.3   Transvaginal ultrasound image of endometrial hyperplasia.

women who are not sexually active or who are trying to conceive

2. CHC: pills, patches, contraceptive ring
3. Progestogen-only contraception (POC): pills, contraceptive injection, implant, Levonorgestrel intrauterine system (IUS)[1]

Combined hormonal contraception and progestogen-only contraception

All clinicians prescribing contraception should be aware of the Faculty of Sexual and Reproductive Healthcare UK medical eligibility criteria[12] (FSRH UKMEC) and method-specific guidelines. (See Table 19.2 for advantages and disadvantages of hormonal contraceptive methods in PCOS).

Table 19.2

Advantages and Disadvantages of Hormonal Contraceptive Methods in PCOS		
Contraception	**Advantages**	**Disadvantages**
Combined hormonal contraception (CHC)	Contraceptive cover Endometrial protection Antiandrogenic benefits Regular bleeding mimicking normal menstrual cycle	Higher contraceptive failure rate as user dependent Increased risk of venous thromboembolism (VTE) (See Table 19.3)/ stroke/breast cancer/ cervical cancer Multiple contraindications e.g. Raised body mass index/blood pressure/ VTE/cardiovascular risk factors
Dianette® (containing cyproterone acetate–not licensed for contraception alone) or Yasmin® (containing drospirenone)	Increased antiandrogenic benefits	Increased risk of VTE (See Table 19.3)
Combined oral contraceptive pill with low dose of oestrogen containing levonorgestrel or norethisterone	Lowest risk of VTE (See Table 19.3)	

Table 19.2

Advantages and Disadvantages of Different Contraceptive Methods—cont'd		
Contraception	**Advantages**	**Disadvantages**
Progestogen-only pill	Contraceptive cover Endometrial protection	May exacerbate androgenic symptoms Irregular bleeding Higher contraceptive failure rate as user dependent
Implant	Contraceptive cover Lower contraceptive failure rate Endometrial protection Lasts for 3 years	May exacerbate androgenic symptoms Irregular bleeding
Depo-Medroxyprogesterone Acetate (DMPA) Depo-Provera® or Sayana®Press	Contraceptive cover Lower contraceptive failure rate Endometrial protection	May exacerbate androgenic symptoms Delay to return of fertility up to 1 year Weight gain Requires injection every 3/12 Irregular bleeding Reduced bone mineral density
Levonorgestrel Intrauterine System e.g. Mirena®	Contraceptive cover Lower contraceptive failure rate Endometrial protection Lasts for 5 years	May exacerbate androgenic symptoms Irregular bleeding

Other treatments

Hirsutism
- Vaniqua Cream (13.9% eflornithine)
- Nonpharmacologic methods of hair removal – shaving, waxing, plucking, bleaching, electrolysis and laser hair removal[14]

Acne
- Topical retinoid or benzoyl peroxide (Retinoids are teratogenic and should be avoided in pregnancy. Retinoids should only be prescribed with adequate contraception.)
- Oral antibiotics[15]

Alopecia: Women with alopecia should be referred to specialist care for management with antiandrogens

Table 19.3

Combined Hormonal Contraception and Venous Thromboembolism Risk[3]

	Background risk in women not using CHC and not pregnant	COCs containing: Levonorgestrel, Norethisterone or Norgestimate	COCs containing: Desogestrel, Gestodene, Drospirenone or Cyproterone acetate Transdermal patch (Evra®) Vaginal ring (NuvaRing®)	CHC containing Etonogestrel (combined vaginal ring) or Norelgestromin (combined transdermal patch)	Pregnancy
Risk of venous thromboembolism in a year	2/10,000	5–7/10,000	9–12/10,000	6-12/10,000	29/10,000

COC, Combined oral contraception

Metformin: A biguanide, an insulin-sensitising drug that decreases gluconeogenesis and increases peripheral utilisation of glucose. It is licensed for use in patients with type 2 diabetes mellitus (T2DM); however, is used 'off licence' in patients with PCOS for symptomatic management.[16]

KEY POINTS

- Polycystic ovary syndrome (PCOS) is a common and complex syndrome with a large spectrum of clinical symptoms and wider-reaching systemic implications

- The mainstay of management is screening for associated conditions such as endometrial hyperplasia and impaired glucose tolerance, lifestyle and weight loss advice, endometrial protection, treatment with hormonal contraception and management of acne and hirsutism

- Hormonal contraception can be challenging because of the misconceptions and comorbidities associated with PCOS

References

1. Graham A, Hamoda H. Treatment of Polycystic Ovarian Syndrome in Primary Care. Prescriber. 2016;27(11):36-45

2. RCOG. Long-term consequences of polycystic ovary syndrome. Royal College of Obstetricians and Gynaecologists; 2014. www.rcog.org.uk. [Free full-text accessed 28/4/21: https://www.rcog.org.uk/en/guidelines-research-services/guidelines/gtg33/]

3. March WA, Moore VM, Wilson KJ, Phillips DI, Norman RJ, Davies M J. The prevalence of polycystic ovarian syndrome in a community sample assessed under contrasting diagnostic criteria. Hum Reprod 2010;25:544–551. Accessed 28/4/21.

4. NICE. Clinical knowledge summary polycystic ovary syndrome. National Institute for Clinical Excellence; 2013. www.nice.org.uk. [Free full-text (http://cks.nice.org.uk/polycystic-ovary-syndrome)]

5. Baskind NE, Balen AH. Hypothalamic-pituitary, ovarian and adrenal contributions to polycystic ovary syndrome. Best Pract Res Clin Obstet Gynaecol. 2016 Nov;37:80-97. doi: 10.1016/j.bpobgyn.2016.03.005. Epub 2016 Apr 1. PMID: 27137106.

6. Ehrmann DA. Polycystic ovary syndrome. N Engl J Med 2005;352(12)1223–1236.

7. Costello M, Shrestha B, Eden J, Sjoblom P, Johnson N. Insulin-sensitising drugs versus the combined oral contraceptive pill for hirsutism, acne and risk of diabetes, cardiovascular disease, and endometrial cancer in polycystic ovary syndrome. Cochrane Database Syst Rev. 2007 Jan 24;(1):CD005552. doi: 10.1002/14651858. CD005552.pub2. Update in: Cochrane Database Syst Rev. 2020 Aug 13;8:CD005552. PMID: 17253562.

8. Balen AH, Conway GS, Kaltsas G, Techatrasak K, Manning PJ, West C, Jacobs HS. Polycystic ovary syndrome: the spectrum of the disorder in 1741 patients. Hum Reprod. 1995 Aug;10(8):2107-11. doi: 10.1093/oxfordjournals.humrep.a136243. PMID: 8567849. [Abstract accessed 28/4/21: https://pubmed.ncbi.nlm.nih.gov/8567849/]

9. Rotterdam ESHRE/ASRM-Sponsored PCOS Consensus Workshop Group. Revised 2003 consensus on diagnostic criteria and long-term health risks related to polycystic

ovary syndrome. Fertil Steril 2004;81(1):19–25. [Abstract (http://www.ncbi.nlm.nih.gov/pubmed/14711538)] Accessed 28/4/21.

10. International evidence based guideline for the assessment and management of polycystic ovary syndrome. Copyright Monash University, Melbourne Australia 2018. [Full text accessed 28/4/21: https://www.monash.edu/__data/assets/pdf_file/0004/1412644/PCOS_Evidence-Based-Guidelines_20181009.pdf]

11. Mansour D. Safer prescribing of therapeutic norethisterone for women at risk of venous thromboembolism. J Fam Plann Reprod Health Care 2012;38:148–149.

12. Faculty of Sexual & Reproductive Health. UK medical eligibility criteria for contraceptive use. 2016. www.fsrh.org.uk. Accessed 28/4/2021: URL https://www.fsrh.org/standards-and-guidance/uk-medical-eligibility-criteria-for-contraceptive-use-ukmec/

13. FSRH. FSRH Guideline Combined hormonal contraception. 2020. [Free full text accessed 28.4.21: https://www.fsrh.org/standards-and-guidance/documents/combined-hormonal-contraception/]

14. NICE. Clinical knowledge summary – hirsutism. National Institute for Clinical Excellence; 2014. www.nice.org.uk [Free full-text (http://cks.nice.org.uk/hirsutism)] Accessed 28/4/21

15. NICE. Clinical knowledge summary – acne vulgaris. National Institute for Clinical Excellence; 2014. www.nice.org.uk. Accessed 28/4/21: (http://cks.nice.org.uk/topics/acne-vulgaris/

16. NICE. British national formulary (BNF 2018). 2018. https://bnf.nice.org.uk/. (Accessed August 2018).

Contraception for Women with Obesity

ANNETTE THWAITES • USHA KUMAR

Case

Shamilla is a 25-year-old woman with a body mass index (BMI) of 35 kg/m^2 (weight 89 kg, height 1.6 m). She has been overweight since childhood and used the contraceptive injection 'on and off' as a teen. She has also had the contraceptive implant once in the past but had this taken out after a few months, as she was worried it was making her put on weight. She has no children and has had two terminations of pregnancy. She had a gastric band fitted almost 2 years ago when her weight had peaked at BMI over 40 kg/m^2 and has subsequently lost 20 kg. She has no other significant medical history. She feels motivated to continue her weight loss and wants to have children in the future. She attends the sexual health clinic requesting emergency and ongoing contraception because she has a new boyfriend. She has been using condoms but had unprotected sexual intercourse last night. She has had no other sex this menstrual cycle.

You discuss the importance of preconception health and the increased risks with pregnancy in obese women, as well as those during the initial weight-loss phase, post bariatric surgery. You counsel Shamilla that the most effective long-acting reversible contraceptive (LARC) methods should be considered until her weight has stabilized. You also advise Shamilla that the effectiveness of oral emergency contraceptive pills may be reduced because of her BMI and bariatric surgery but that she is eligible for the most effective form of emergency contraception, the intrauterine device (IUD), which can also be used for ongoing contraception. With regard to her options for ongoing contraception, you counsel her that, although there is limited evidence regarding the efficacy of oral contraceptive pills in women post bariatric surgery, this could potentially be reduced and also has relatively higher typical-use failure rates. You discuss the association of depo-medroxyprogesterone acetate (DMPA) with weight gain but reassure her that there is no evidence of such association for any other methods. You explain that, at her current weight, the use of combined hormonal methods would not be recommended (UK medical eligibility criteria [UKMEC] 3)[1] because of increased risk of venous thromboembolism (VTE). You encourage and support her plans for sustained weight loss. She opts for an emergency IUD fitting today and also accepts the offer of a sexual health screen.

Introduction and epidemiology

Increasing obesity is a pressing national and worldwide public health issue. For adults aged over 20 years, the World Health Organization (WHO) defines 'overweight' as a BMI greater than or equal to 25 kg/m^2; and 'obesity' is a BMI greater than or equal to 30 kg/m^2.[2] In 2016, 40% of women globally were overweight and of these 15% were obese.[3] In England, 6 out of 10 women aged 16 years and over are overweight or obese (59%); more than one in four women is obese (29%), and prevalence continues to increase.[4]

Obese women are at increased risk, compared with women of normal weight, of a wide range of other comorbidities, including VTE, hypertension, dyslipidaemias, type 2 diabetes, cardiovascular disease, stroke, and some cancers (including breast and endometrial cancer).[5] They also face increased risks in pregnancy of maternal and infant mortality and morbidity with higher rates of gestational hypertension, diabetes, preeclampsia, thromboembolism, prolonged labour, caesarean delivery, anaesthetic complications, wound infections, and postpartum haemorrhage together with adverse foetal outcomes, such as growth restriction, neural tube defects, miscarriage, stillbirth, and neonatal death.[6,7,8] Importantly, maternal obesity also negatively affects the health of future generations with predisposition to obesity and diabetes in offspring in later life.[5]

Clinical presentation

An awareness of the associated health risks and effective preconception care are vital for women with obesity. Despite an association between obesity and subfertility, and misconceptions held by women regarding their fertility, many obese women conceive without difficulty, and provision of effective contraception is key to avoiding unplanned pregnancy. Women with obesity may present in a wide variety of clinical settings, and healthcare professionals should encourage obese women of reproductive age to lose weight before conceiving, and to use contraception while aiming for a target weight.[8] They may present for contraception to their general practitioners, walk-in sexual health services and as referrals into specialist contraception clinics. Weight should be regularly measured during contraception consultations and advice given on weight and lifestyle factors to help women optimise their weight before pregnancy.[9] Contraceptive needs of women with obesity should also be addressed in other settings, including abortion, subfertility, recurrent miscarriage, diabetic clinics and bariatric surgical assessment and follow-up.

Contraception

Contraception safety

For women with obesity with no co-existent medical conditions, all progestogen-only and intrauterine contraceptive methods are categorised as UKMEC 1, that is, unrestricted use. In contrast, oestrogen-containing contraception is UKMEC 2 or 3, depending on BMI (see Table 20.1). The restrictions are primarily caused by increased cardiovascular risks from exogenous oestrogen, including VTE, acute myocardial infarction and stroke. The risk for VTE in obese women is double that of women of normal weight and rises as BMI increases over 30 kg/m^2, increasing further with BMI over 35 kg/m^2.[5]

However, if a woman with obesity has other risk factors for cardiovascular disease (CVD), the UKMEC categories are increased across all hormonal methods. The levonorgestrel-releasing intrauterine system, implant and progestogen-only pill (POP) are UKMEC 2 (the advantages of using the method generally outweigh the theoretical or proven risks); DMPA and combined hormonal contraception are UKMEC 3 (the theoretical or proven risks usually outweigh the advantages of using the method). When discussing contraceptive options with a woman who is overweight or obese, clinicians should counsel as to the relevant potential weight-related risks.[10]

Table 20.1[1]

United Kingdom Medical Eligibility Criteria Summary Table Hormonal and Intrauterine Contraception for Women with Obesity and Cardiovascular Disease						
Condition	**Cu-IUD**	**LNG-IUS**	**IMP**	**DMPA**	**POP**	**CHC**
Obesity						
BMI ≥30–34 kg/m²	1	1	1	1	1	2
BMI ≥35 kg/m²	1	1	1	1	1	3
Cardiovascular Disease (CVD)						
Multiple risk factors for CVD (such as smoking, diabetes, hypertension, obesity and dyslipidaemias)	1	2	2	3	2	3

BMI, Body mass index; *CHC*, combined hormonal contraception; *Cu-IUD*, copper intrauterine device; *DMPA*, depo-medroxyprogesterone acetate; *IMP*, progestogen-only implant; *LNG-IUS*, levonorgestrel-releasing intrauterine system; *POP*, progestogen-only pill. Reproduced under licence from FSRH. Copyright ©Faculty of Sexual and Reproductive Healthcare 2006 to 2016.

Contraception efficacy

Association between obesity and contraception failure has been proposed but is difficult to analyse and differentiate between method failure and user failure.[6] Obesity does not increase the risk of failure of most contraceptive methods.

- Effectiveness of intrauterine methods is not known to be affected by weight.
- Whereas the Summary of Product Characteristics for the Nexplanon® implant states theoretical potential reduction in the duration of contraceptive efficacy for women who weigh ≥150 kg and consideration of early replacement,[11] recent Faculty of Sexual & Reproductive Healthcare (FSRH) guidance recommends that there is currently no direct evidence to support a need for earlier implant replacement and that the licensed duration of Nexplanon® use of 3 years applies to women of all weight categories.[5]
- No increased risk of pregnancy has been demonstrated in progestogen-only injectable users with higher body weight, although data are limited in women with a BMI of 40 kg/m² or more.[12]

- Whereas most evidence suggests no association between weight and combined oral contraceptive or combined vaginal ring effectiveness,[5] the Summary of Product Characteristics for the combined patch specifies that contraceptive efficacy may be decreased in women weighing 90 kg or more,[13] and current FSRH guidance states additional precautions or an alternative method should be advised.[5,14]

- Available evidence suggests that effectiveness of POP is not affected by body weight or BMI. Increased dosage of the POP is not recommended for women who are overweight/obese.[15]

- Current FSRH guidance on emergency contraception states that BMI over 26 kg/m^2 or weight over 70 kg could reduce the effectiveness of levonorgestrel emergency contraception (LNG-EC), and that double-dose (3 mg) LNG can be used if an IUD/ulipristal acetate emergency contraception (UPA-EC) is not suitable. Limited evidence also suggests that UPA-EC could potentially be less effective for women over 85 kg or with a BMI greater than 30 kg/m^2.[16]

Contraception and weight gain

Many women believe that weight gain is a common side effect of contraception.[10] This in turn may deter obese women from initiating certain hormonal methods. Perceived weight gain is also one of the leading reasons for discontinuing contraception[5,6] and may be a particular concern for women already overweight. However, adult women tend to gain weight over time during the reproductive years regardless of contraceptive use, most likely because of genetic, environmental and lifestyle factors,[5] and clinicians should reassure women that there is currently no conclusive evidence demonstrating a causative effect of contraception on weight gain. There is, however, an association between DMPA use and weight gain, particularly in women under 18 years of age with a BMI of 30 kg/m^2 or more,[12] and women who gain more than 5% of their baseline body weight in the first 6 months of DMPA use are likely to experience continued weight gain.

Contraception and bariatric surgery

National Institute for Health and Care Excellence guidelines recommend that bariatric or weight-loss surgery be considered when

Table 20.2[1]

United Kingdom Medical Eligibility Criteria Summary Table Hormonal and Intrauterine Contraception following Bariatric Surgery						
Condition	Cu-IUD	LNG-IUS	IMP	DMPA	POP	CHC
History of bariatric surgery						
With BMI <30 kg/m^2	1	1	1	1	1	1
With BMI ≥30–34 kg/m^2	1	1	1	1	1	2
With BMI ≥35 kg/m^2	1	1	1	1	1	3

BMI, Body mass index; *CHC*, combined hormonal contraception; *Cu-IUD*, copper intrauterine device; *DMPA*, depo-medroxyprogesterone acetate; *IMP*, progestogen-only implant; *LNG-IUS*, levonorgestrel-releasing intrauterine system; *POP*, progestogen-only pill. Reproduced under licence from FSRH. Copyright ©Faculty of Sexual and Reproductive Healthcare 2006 to 2016.

the BMI is 40 kg/m^2 or more, or for those with a BMI between 35 and 40 kg/m^2 in the presence of other co-morbidities and where other non-surgical methods have proven unsuccessful.[17] Bariatric surgery may be restrictive, aiming to reduce calorie intake by reducing gastric capacity (e.g., laparoscopic adjustable gastric banding, silastic ring gastroplasty, vertical banded gastroplasty and sleeve gastrectomy) and/or malabsorptive (e.g., biliopancreatic diversion and Roux-en-Y gastric bypass).[18] Some 80% of women requesting bariatric surgery are of reproductive age.[19]

The safety of different contraceptive methods post bariatric surgery aligns with the general weight category (see Table 20.2). However, the UKMEC states that women within 2 years post bariatric surgery should be advised to consider the most effective LARC methods,[1] and that sole use of barrier and user-dependent methods may not be appropriate because of their relatively higher typical-use failure rates. This is to avoid pregnancy while still in an initial weight loss phase and any concurrent postoperative complications, which may pose a significant health risk.[5,18] Bariatric surgical procedures that result in a malabsorptive effect may also decrease the effectiveness of oral contraceptive methods in the longer term.

Table 20.3 summarises the benefits and risks associated with different methods for women with obesity.

Table 20.3

Benefits and Risks of Contraceptive Methods		
Type	**Benefits**	**Risks/Disadvantages/ Considerations**
Cu-intrauterine device (Cu-IUD)	• Highly effective for 5 or 10 years • Can be used as emergency and on-going contraception • No association between IUC use and weight gain • Effectiveness of IUC is not known to be affected by weight or BMI	• May be technically more difficult insertion (e.g., difficulty in visualising cervix, assessing size/ direction of uterus) • May require specialist setting (e.g., access to ultrasound, supportive gynaecology couch, range of specula sizes, large blood pressure cuff)
Intrauterine systems (IUS)	• Highly effective for 3 or 5 years • No association between IUC use and weight gain • Effectiveness of IUC is not known to be affected by weight or BMI • Also used as treatment for endometrial hyperplasia (Obesity is a risk factor for endometrial hyperplasia and endometrial cancer)	• May be technically more difficult insertion (e.g., difficulty in visualising cervix, assessing size/direction of uterus) • May require specialist setting (e.g., access to ultrasound, supportive gynaecology couch, range of specula sizes, large blood pressure cuff)
Nexplanon® implant	• Highly effective for 3 years • No evidence suggesting a causal association between implant use and weight gain	

Continued

Table 20.3

Benefits and Risks of Contraceptive Methods—cont'd		
Type	**Benefits**	**Risks/Disadvantages/ Considerations**
Depo-Medroxyprogesterone Acetate (DMPA) injection	• Highly effective • Effectiveness of DMPA is not known to be affected by weight or BMI	• If obesity is one of multiple risk factors for cardiovascular disease, then UKMEC 3 • Associated with weight gain, particularly in women under 18 years of age with a BMI of 30 kg/m² or more[12] • If ability to administer an IM injection because of body habitus is doubtful, then the deltoid muscle in the upper arm or subcutaneous DMPA (Sayana Press®) could be used
Progestogen only pill (POP)	• Medium effectiveness as user dependent • No association between POP use and weight gain • No association between weight/BMI and POP effectiveness	• Medications that induce diarrhoea and/or vomiting (e.g., Orlistat, laxatives) may reduce the effectiveness of POP • Not recommended as sole form of contraception in first 2 years post bariatric surgery • The effectiveness of oral contraception in women who have had bariatric surgery could be reduced. Women undergoing bariatric surgery with a significant malabsorption component should preferentially consider non-oral methods

Table 20.3

Benefits and Risks of Contraceptive Methods—cont'd

Type	Benefits	Risks/Disadvantages/Considerations
Combined hormonal contraception (CHC)	• Medium effectiveness as user dependent • No association between CHC use and weight gain • Most evidence suggests no association between weight/BMI and COC or ring effectiveness[5]	• CHC is UKMEC 2 for BMI $\geq$ 30–34 kg/m^2, and UKMEC 3 for BMI $\geq$35 kg/m^2 • Contraceptive efficacy of the patch may be decreased in women weighing $\geq$90 kg[13] • Medications that induce diarrhoea and/or vomiting (e.g., Orlistat, laxatives) may reduce the effectiveness of COC • Not recommended as sole form of contraception in first 2 years post bariatric surgery • The effectiveness of oral contraception in women who have had bariatric surgery could be reduced. Women undergoing bariatric surgery with a significant malabsorption component should preferentially consider non-oral methods
Emergency oral contraception		• BMI >26 kg/m^2 or weight >70 kg could reduce the effectiveness of LNG-EC. Consider UPA or double-dose (3 mg) LNG[16] • The effectiveness of oral emergency contraception in women who have had bariatric surgery could be reduced

Continued

Table 20.3

Benefits and Risks of Contraceptive Methods—cont'd		
Type	**Benefits**	**Risks/Disadvantages/ Considerations**
Barrier methods	• Condoms provide protection against sexually transmitted infections	• Low effectiveness with higher typical-use failure rates • Not recommended as sole form of contraception in first 2 years post bariatric surgery • During period of significant weight loss (e.g., post bariatric surgery), diaphragm may no longer fit, and sizing would need to be checked before restarting this method
Laparoscopic sterilisation	• Permanent method	• Increased risk of anaesthetic and surgical complications and failed procedure

BMI, Body mass index; *COC*, combined oral contraception; *IUC*, intrauterine contraception; *LNG-EC*, levonorgestrel for emergency contraception; *UPA*, ulipristal acetate emergency contraception.

KEY POINTS

- Pregnancy in women with obesity is associated with increased risk of maternal and infant mortality and morbidity

- Healthcare professionals should ensure women with obesity are aware of these risks and have access to effective methods of contraception, weight loss support, preconception advice and maternity care

- Obesity may present an unacceptable health risk for the use of combined and injectable hormonal contraceptive methods depending on a woman's body mass index and other risk factors for venous thromboembolism and cardiovascular disease

- Obesity does not increase the risk of failure of most contraceptive methods

- Women undergoing bariatric surgery should be advised to avoid pregnancy for 2 years post surgery and consider use of the most effective long-acting reversible contraception methods

- Oral contraception is not recommended in women who have had bariatric surgical procedures with a significant malabsorption component because of a higher failure risk

References

1. Faculty of Sexual & Reproductive Healthcare. UK medical eligibility criteria for contraceptive use. 2016. https://www.fsrh.org/standards-and-guidance/external/ukmec-2016-digital-version/.
2. World Health Organization Regional Office for Europe: Body mass index – BMI 2015. www.euro.who.int/en/health-topics/disease-prevention/nutrition/a-healthy-lifestyle/body-mass-index-bmi (Accessed 28 March 2021).
3. World Health Organization. Factsheet No. 311 – Obesity and Overweight. September 2004. Geneva. http://www.who.int/news-room/fact-sheets/detail/obesity-and-overweight (Accessed 28 March 2021).
4. https://digital.nhs.uk/data-and-information/publications/statistical/statistics-on-obesity-physical-activity-and-diet/england-2020/part-3-adult-obesity-copy.
5. Faculty of Sexual & Reproductive Healthcare. FSRH guideline overweight, obesity and contraception. 2019. https://www.fsrh.org/standards-and-guidance/documents/fsrh-clinical-guideline-overweight-obesity-and-contraception/.
6. Mahmood T, Arulkumaran S, editors. Obesity: a ticking time bomb for reproductive health. ISBN: 978-0124160453, Hardback, 670 pages, Elsevier; 2012.
7. The Confidential Enquiry into Maternal and Child Health (CEMACH). Saving Mothers' Lives: Reviewing Maternal Deaths to Make Motherhood Safer – 2003–2005. The Seventh Report on Confidential Enquiries into Maternal Deaths in the United Kingdom. Lewis G, editor. London: CEMACH; 2007.
8. Ramsay JE, Greer I, Sattar N. Obesity and reproduction. BMJ 2006;333:1159–1162.
9. Royal College of Obstetricians and Gynaecologists. Care of women with obesity in pregnancy. 2018. https://www.rcog.org.uk/en/guidelines-research-services/guidelines/management-of-women-with-obesity-in-pregnancy/.
10. Faculty of Sexual & Reproductive Healthcare. Clinical effectiveness unit. Statement on weight and contraception. 2017. https://www.fsrh.org/news/ceu-statement-on-weight-and-contraception-how-do-they-influence/.
11. Electronic Medicines Compendium. Summary of Product Characteristics: Nexplanon 68mg implant for subdermal use. 8 December 2014. http://www.medicines.org.uk/emc/medicine/23824.
12. Faculty of Sexual & Reproductive Healthcare. Progestogen-only contraceptive injection. 2014. https://www.fsrh.org/standards-and-guidance/documents/cec-ceu-guidance-injectables-dec-2014/.
13. Electronic Medicines Compendium . Summary of Product Characteristics: Evra transdermal patch. 2017. https://www.medicines.org.uk/emc/medicine/12124/SPC/Evra++transdermal+patch/.
14. Faculty of Sexual & Reproductive Healthcare. Combined Hormonal Contraception. 2019 (updated February 2019). https://www.fsrh.org/standards-and-guidance/documents/combined-hormonal-contraception/.
15. Faculty of Sexual & Reproductive Healthcare. Progestogen-only pills. 2015 (updated February 2019). https://www.fsrh.org/standards-and-guidance/documents/cec-ceu-guidance-pop-mar-2015/.

16. Faculty of Sexual & Reproductive Healthcare. Emergency contraception. 2017. https://www.fsrh.org/standards-and-guidance/current-clinical-guidance/emergency-contraception/.

17. National Institute for Health and Care Excellence. Obesity: guidance on the prevention of overweight and obesity in adults and children. NICE clinical guideline 43. Manchester: NICE; 2006. https://www.nice.org.uk/ guidance/cg43/resources/guidance-obesity-pdf].

18. Royal College of Obstetricians and Gynaecologists. The role of bariatric surgery in improving reproductive health scientific impact paper No. 17. 2015. https://www.rcog.org.uk/globalassets/documents/guidelines/scientific-impact-papers/sip_17.pdf.

19. The UK National bariatric surgery registry: second registry report. 2014. http://www.bomss.org.uk/wp-content/uploads/2014/04/Extract_from_the_NBSR_2014_Report.pdf.

Contraception for Women with Eating Disorders

ANNETTE THWAITES • USHA KUMAR

Case

Emma is 17 years old and is studying for A-levels. She attends the sexual health clinic requesting contraception, as she has a new boyfriend. She says her periods have been irregular for a while and that she has not had one for a few months now. Her body mass index (BMI) is 19 kg/m² (weight 45 kg, height 1.53 m). She was seen in the clinic a year ago for emergency contraception and her BMI then was 22 kg/m² (weight 54 kg). On direct questioning, she says that she has recently been referred by her general practitioner (GP) to a psychiatrist to discuss her eating and weight loss and is waiting for her first appointment. Emma is shocked and upset when her pregnancy test is positive today. She has had two casual sexual partners in the last year and did not use any contraception because she thought she could not get pregnant when she was not getting regular periods. She has not discussed fertility or contraception with her GP.

You advise Emma of the pregnancy options, and she is very sure that she wants a surgical termination of pregnancy. You help Emma to arrange her procedure and advise her that she will need effective contraception afterwards even if she continues to be amenorrhoeic. You advise that the most effective long-acting reversible contraception (LARC) methods can be fitted at the time of her procedure and give her written and verbal information on all methods. She has used the combined oral contraceptive pill before, but as she admits to self-inducing vomiting sometimes, you explain that oral methods may well be less effective for her. She later opts for the implant. You also perform a sexually transmitted infection screen for her today. Emma will need preop investigations, including urea & electrolytes, magnesium, calcium, phosphate, liver function tests, full blood count, and electrocardiogram and anaesthetic review if there are any abnormalities.

Introduction and epidemiology

Eating disorders are serious psychiatric conditions with physical, psychologic and social consequences. They are categorised by distorted self-body image and abnormal attitudes and behaviour towards eating and are diagnosed clinically, according to the DSM 5 criteria.[1] Anorexia nervosa (anorexia) and bulimia nervosa (bulimia) are the most well-known types, but binge eating disorder and other specified feeding or eating disorder (OSFED) are the most common.[2] Anorexia involves deliberate dietary restriction, leading to significantly low body weight and an intense fear of weight gain. In contrast, women with bulimia are usually of normal or above normal weight and the disorder is characterized by recurrent episodes of binge eating and inappropriate compensatory behaviour to prevent weight gain, such as self-induced vomiting or misuse of laxatives. Binge eating disorders are not associated with the recurrent use of inappropriate compensatory behaviour, and OSFED includes other eating disorders that do not meet the full diagnostic criteria for any other specified eating disorders.

The true prevalence of eating disorders is difficult to establish, as available statistics relate to those receiving care and so do not reflect the undiagnosed in the community. Annual UK incidence rates have been estimated at around 63 per 100,000 women of all ages and are highest among 15- to 19-year-olds at around 165 per 100,000.[3] However, as these figures are likely to be underestimates, we can assume eating disorders are not uncommon in adolescent women.

Clinical presentation: signs and symptoms

Women with eating disorders often have a tendency to conceal their behaviours and resist healthcare professional input, and outcomes are poor, particularly in anorexia, if women do not receive effective treatment in the first three years.[4] It is therefore important for clinicians to retain a high level of suspicion for the presence of eating disorders in patients, talk directly to women about their weight and eating patterns, and be able to refer on to specialists for further assessment and management.

Women with eating disorders may present to sexual and reproductive health care or gynaecology services with oligo- or amenorrhoea, fertility concerns or unplanned pregnancy. They may also present in the context of sexual risk taking or sexual abuse. Clinicians should be alert to the possibility of underlying eating disorders, especially if a patient has a low BMI or menstrual disturbance. Subtle signs may be apparent during consultations: for example, Russell's sign, marking across the knuckles and dorsum of hand from self-induced vomiting; swollen parotid and submandibular glands or erosion of anterior tooth enamel secondary to repeated vomiting; and lanugo, fine downy hair on the arms, chest, back and face as a means of maintaining body temperature when fat stores are depleted.

It must be remembered that not all eating disorders result in low weight and, as in our case study, women of short stature can lose more than 20% of their body weight and still remain in the normal range for BMI. Menstrual disturbance can also precede weight loss, so this symptom should always prompt consideration of an eating disorder, regardless of weight. Patients are often routinely weighed and measured when prescribing contraception, and trends can be helpful to aid diagnosis.

Contraception

Women with eating disorders require effective contraception, despite amenorrhoea and anovulation being common in this population, as it is impossible to predict when ovulation may occur.[5] The extent of any disruption to fertility in women with eating disorders is still unknown and remains an active area of research. Moreover, for those who conceive when they are underweight, there is an increased risk of adverse pregnancy outcomes, including intrauterine growth restriction and preterm birth.[6,7] Postponement of conception until the eating disorder is in remission is therefore recommended.[5] Clinicians should therefore ensure that women with eating disorders are correctly informed as to their need for effective contraception and advised as to specific safety and efficacy concerns of each method.

Table 21.1 highlights the benefits and risks associated with each method. Intrauterine methods and the contraceptive implant are the most effective contraceptive methods[8] and should be first line in those women who need to avoid pregnancy until in remission.[5] There are no absolute contraindications to these LARC methods in this group of women, but the table below highlights when extra care should be taken. Specific considerations related

Table 21.1

Benefits and Risks of Contraceptive Methods		
Type	**Benefits**	**Risks and Disadvantages**
Cu-intrauterine device (Cu-IUD)	• Highly effective • Unaffected by vomiting or laxatives	• Increased risk of vasovagal reaction at insertion if bradycardia or hypotension, secondary to eating disorder, or if has not eaten on day of insertion • Increased risk of prolonged QT interval with anorexia is a UKMEC 3 for initiation of intrauterine contraception[11] and will need liaison with a cardiologist • If short uterine cavity, secondary to anorexia in adolescence, may necessitate small device
Intrauterine systems (IUS)	• Highly effective • Unaffected by vomiting or laxatives	• May be associated with hormonal side effects (e.g., breast tenderness, bloating) which may be less acceptable to this group • Increased risk of vasovagal reaction at insertion if secondary bradycardia, hypotension or has not eaten on day of insertion • Increased risk of prolonged QT interval with anorexia (UKMEC 3[11]) • If short uterine cavity, secondary to anorexia in adolescence, may necessitate small device
Nexplanon® implant	• Highly effective • Unaffected by vomiting or laxatives	• May be associated with hormonal side effects (e.g., breast tenderness, bloating) which may be less acceptable to this group • Potential increased risk of deep insertion if low BMI.[13]; experienced fitter recommended • Implants may be more visible in thin arms
Depo-medroxyprogesterone acetate (DMPA) injection	• Highly effective • Unaffected by vomiting or laxatives	• Associated with weight gain • Associated with reduced bone mineral density (BMD)

Table 21.1

Benefits and Risks of Contraceptive Methods—cont'd		
Type	**Benefits**	**Risks and Disadvantages**
Progestogen only pill (POP)	• Medium effectiveness	• Can be affected by vomiting or laxatives • May be associated with hormonal side effects (e.g., breast tenderness, bloating) which may be less acceptable to this group
Combined hormonal contraception (CHC)	• Medium effectiveness • Patch and ring are unaffected by vomiting or laxatives	• COC can be affected by vomiting or laxatives • May be associated with hormonal side effects (e.g., breast tenderness, bloating) which may be less acceptable to this group • Cyclic bleeding may provide false reassurance of a return to regular menstrual function and recovery

BMI, Body mass index; *COC,* combined oral contraceptives.

to bone mineral density, vomiting and laxative abuse are additionally discussed later.

Bone mineral density

Anorexia and bulimia are known risk factors for osteoporosis, even in women with normal weight. The mechanism is likely multifactorial and poorly understood.[5] Combined hormonal methods have been commonly used in women with anorexia as prophylaxis and treatment for low bone mineral density (BMD), but this is not evidence-based practice.[5] It is possible that oestrogen treatment alone cannot correct the multiple factors (nutritional, other hormonal) contributing to loss of BMD.[9] Women with anorexia should not be reassured that combined hormonal contraception is protective against osteoporosis in the absence of weight gain.[5] Depo-medroxyprogesterone acetate (DMPA) is associated with a small and recoverable reduction in BMD,[8] and because adolescence is a crucial time period for attaining peak BMD,[10] this method is a UK medical eligibility criteria (UKMEC) 2 in women aged less than 18 years.[11] It is therefore not recommended in women with eating disorders at risk of osteoporosis.[10]

Vomiting and laxative abuse

Absorption of oral contraception from the small intestine may be affected by drugs that cause vomiting or severe diarrhoea, or by drugs that alter gut transit.[12] Clinicians should ask women with eating disorders directly whether they are or have ever self-induced vomiting or used laxatives or other drugs to try and lose weight or avoid weight gain. If so, women should be advised to use non-oral methods of contraception. However, if a woman still wishes to use pills, then she must be clearly advised regarding the risk of pill failure and need for a repeat dose and extra precautions if she vomits within 3 hours of pill taking or has severe diarrhoea.[12]

Sexual health

Women with eating disorders should be given the same advice as all women with regard to screening for sexually transmitted infections, condom use and sexual health. Women with anorexia may also experience vaginal dryness and dyspareunia secondary to hypoestrogenism, and use of a lubricant during sex and topical oestrogen may be helpful.[5]

KEY POINTS

- Women with eating disorders can be of normal or above normal body mass index and weight

- Women with eating disorders should be advised of the increased risk of adverse pregnancy outcomes when underweight and advised to delay conception until in remission

- Sexually active women with eating disorders require effective contraception despite menstrual irregularities and oligomenorrhoea/amenorrhoea because it is not possible to predict when ovulation and an unintended pregnancy may occur

- Long-acting reversible contraception methods (intrauterine methods and implant) remain the most effective methods of contraception in this population

- Combined hormonal contraceptives have not been shown to protect bone mineral density in women with anorexia

- Injectable contraceptive methods should be avoided in patients with anorexia and other eating disorders which are a risk factor for osteoporosis

- Non-oral methods should be recommended in women who are self-inducing vomiting or using laxatives

References

1. American Psychiatric Association. Diagnostic and statistical manual of mental disorders: DSM-5. Washington, DC: American Psychiatric Publishing; 2013.
2. NHS Choices. Eating disorders. National Health Service; 2018. https://www.nhs.uk/conditions/eating-disorders/.
3. Micali N, Hagberg KW, Petersen I, Treasure JL. The incidence of eating disorders in the UK in 2000–2009: findings from the General Practice Research Database. BMJ Open 2013;3:e002646.
4. Bould H, Newbegin C, Stewart A, Stein A, Fazel M. Eating disorders in children and young people. BMJ 2017;359:j5245.
5. Faculty of Sexual and Reproductive Healthcare. FSRH CEU statement: contraception for women with eating disorders. June 15, 2018. https://www.fsrh.org/documents/fsrh-ceu-statement-contraception-for-women-with-eating/.
6. Becker AE, Grinspoon SK, Klibanski A, Herzog DB. Eating disorders. N Engl J Med 1999;340:1092-1098.
7. Koubaa S, Hällström T, Lindholm C, Hirschberg AL. Pregnancy and neonatal outcomes in women with eating disorders. Obstet Gynecol 2005;105:255–260.
8. National Institute for Health and Clinical Excellence. Long-acting reversible contraception: the effective and appropriate use of long-acting reversible contraception. National Institute for Health and Clinical Excellence; 2014. https://www.nice.org.uk/guidance/cg30.
9. Klibanski A, Biller BM, Schoenfeld DA, Herzog DB, Saxe VC. The effects of estrogen administration on trabecular bone loss in young women with anorexia nervosa. J Clin Endocrinol Metab 1995;80:898–904.
10. Faculty of Sexual & Reproductive Healthcare. Progestogen-only contraceptive injection. 2014. https://www.fsrh.org/standards-and-guidance/documents/cec-ceu-guidance-injectables-dec-2014/.
11. Faculty of Sexual & Reproductive Healthcare. UK medical eligibility criteria for contraceptive use. 2016. https://www.fsrh.org/standards-and-guidance/external/ukmec-2016-digital- version/.
12. Faculty of Sexual & Reproductive Healthcare. Drug interactions with hormonal contraception. 2017. https://www.fsrh.org/documents/ceu-clinical-guidance-drug-interactions-with-hormonal/.
13. Merck Sharp and Dohme Limited. Letter to healthcare professionals regarding Nexplanon migration. 2016. https://assets.publishing.service.gov.uk/media/576006d640f0b652dd000036/Nexplanon_DHPC_sent_31_May_2016.pdf.

Contraception for Women with Epilepsy

ANNETTE THWAITES • USHA KUMAR

Case

Caroline is 46 years old with long-standing epilepsy. She has two children aged 7 and 11 years. She was well controlled on lamotrigine monotherapy during her two pregnancies but has been taking sodium valproate also for the last 4 years because of an increase in seizures after her most recent delivery, which she feels was triggered by stress and fatigue. She has now been seizure-free for 3 years. She has been married for 20 years and has been using condoms consistently with her husband for the last 7 years. She has no other medical problems; her body mass index (BMI) is 23 kg/m^2, her blood pressure (BP) is 115/89 mm Hg and she is a non-smoker. You take a detailed menstrual history and screen for any menopausal symptoms. Her menstrual periods have become somewhat less frequent and heavier over the last year, and she has recently been experiencing some hot flashes also.

Caroline must be counselled regarding the teratogenicity of sodium valproate and her consequent need for the most effective contraceptive methods. She must also be aware that she will need to continue to use effective contraception until age 55 years, or until 2 years after her last menstrual period, if she experiences menopause aged 50 years (or younger) or until 1 year after her last menstrual period if her menopause occurs after the age of 50 years. She should be informed that lamotrigine, although not an enzyme-inducing drug, interacts with oral contraception. Combined hormonal contraception (CHC) moderately reduces lamotrigine exposure, which can lead to decreased seizure control in the active hormone phase and, conversely, a risk of lamotrigine toxicity in the hormone-free week. Desogestrel may increase lamotrigine levels and adverse effects. Ethinylestradiol in CHC may modestly reduce sodium valproate levels also. Long-acting reversible contraceptive (LARC) methods should therefore be recommended, and the intrauterine system (IUS) may be optimal for her. You outline the additional, non-contraceptive benefits associated with the Mirena® IUS of reduction in menstrual bleeding and potential to be used as the progestogen component of hormone replacement therapy (HRT) if required. She opts for a Mirena® IUS, and you fit this for her today. You offer her a routine sexually transmitted infection screening at the same time, and she accepts this. You inform her that she can rely on this Mirena® IUS for contraception until age 55 years but would need to change it every 5 years if used as HRT.

Introduction and epidemiology

Epilepsy is a heterogeneous condition characterised by an increased predisposition to seizures. The majority of cases are idiopathic, with approximately 30% of patients having a family history of epilepsy.[1] The incidence of new cases is 20 to 30 per 100,000 young women in the United Kingdom every year affecting approximately 0.5% to 1% of women of childbearing age.[2] Many anti-epileptic drugs (AEDs) have teratogenic effects and/or are hepatic enzyme inducers that reduce the effectiveness of some contraceptive methods, including oral emergency contraception. Conversely, some hormonal contraception can affect the levels of some AEDs, affecting seizure control or toxicity levels. Epilepsy and its treatments therefore have important consequences for contraception care.

Epilepsy is the most common neurologic condition in pregnancy.[2] Although most women with epilepsy have good pregnancy outcomes, those with unstable epilepsy or otherwise poor health and those taking specific, high-dose or multiple AEDs are at risk of increased maternal mortality and morbidity.[2,3] The risk of death is increased 10-fold in pregnant women with epilepsy compared with those without the condition[3]; a mortality rate higher than any other pre-existing medical condition. The majority of deaths occurring in pregnant women with epilepsy are classified as sudden unexpected death in epilepsy, with poorly controlled seizures being the main contributory factor.[3] Women with epilepsy are also at increased risk of miscarriage, antepartum haemorrhage, hypertensive disorders, induction of labour, caesarean section, preterm delivery and postpartum haemorrhage compared with the background population.[4] Women taking AEDs are at increased risk of major congenital foetal malformation, and exposure to sodium valproate in particular has an adverse effect on the long-term neurodevelopment of the newborn.[5] Maternal concerns regarding the effects of AEDs on their baby may lead to abrupt discontinuation or reduction in the dose of the AEDs, thereby increasing the woman's risk of seizures and poor outcomes.[5] Therefore women with epilepsy of childbearing age require careful counselling and specialist input with regard to their preconception and obstetric care.

Clinical presentation

Women with epilepsy may present to general practitioners and specialist neurology services. They are also commonly seen in walk-in and specialist contraception services and antenatal obstetric clinics. Healthcare professionals in these settings need to be aware of the increased risks to women with epilepsy and those taking AEDs and prioritise their contraceptive needs. Counselling should be tailored to the individual, including current and potential treatment regimens and pregnancy planning. Optimal seizure control should be achieved wherever possible before conception, particularly for women and girls with generalised tonic–clonic seizures. However, potential teratogenic and other adverse effects of AEDs must be considered, lowest effective dose used and polytherapy avoided if possible.[5] Preconception counselling should also address good general health (e.g., exercise, diet, smoking, alcohol), and women with epilepsy should also be advised to take high-dose, 5 mg/day folic acid before conception until at least the end of the first trimester to reduce the incidence of major congenital malformation.[5]

Pregnant women with epilepsy should be seen as early as possible by a neurologist specialising in epilepsy. These women require shared obstetric and neurologist care throughout their pregnancy also.[6] Women with epilepsy should be reassured that most will have normal healthy babies and the risk of congenital malformations is low if they are not exposed to AEDs periconception.[5] Women with generalised tonic–clonic seizures should be informed that the foetus may be at higher relative risk of harm during a seizure, although the absolute risk remains very low and may depend on seizure frequency. Women with focal, absence and myoclonic seizures do not have increased risks in pregnancy unless associated with secondary trauma, for example, falls. Ongoing obstetric care is recommended, and pregnant women taking AEDs may be offered earlier or additional ultrasound scans to screen for structural anomalies.[5] The risk of seizures during labour is low, but delivery in an obstetric unit is still recommended. Immediate postnatal contraception for women with epilepsy should also be considered antenatally and may be appropriate.

Contraception

There is some evidence that women with epilepsy, and those on AEDs, have lower fertility rates than women without epilepsy and higher rates of anovulatory cycles, irregular menstrual bleeding or oligomenorrhea/amenorrhea.[7,8] However, the reduction in fertility in this group is thought to be small, and it is estimated that approximately 50% of all pregnancies in women with epilepsy are unplanned.[8]

All contraceptive methods considered in the UK medical eligibility criteria (UKMEC) 2016 are categorised UKMEC 1 for women with epilepsy[9] (see Table 22.1), and there is no conclusive evidence that hormonal contraception aggravates epileptic seizures.[8]

However, it must be stressed that UKMEC categories relate to safety, *not* efficacy, and interactions with a woman's current or proposed therapeutic regimen may well lead to strong recommendations regarding method selection. A universal principle when managing women and girls with epilepsy should be the provision of consistent, effective contraception to avoid unplanned pregnancy. This is of even greater clinical concern in women taking teratogenic AEDs when LARC methods should be strongly recommended. Enzyme-inducing AEDs (EIAEDs) can reduce the efficacy of oral contraceptives (Combined oral contraception and, progestogen-only pills), transdermal patches, vaginal ring, progestogen-only implants and emergency contraceptive pills. Other drug interactions with non-enzyme-inducing AEDs, for example, lamotrigine (see later), may also have a negative effect on seizure control. Intrauterine and injectable LARC methods of contraception are not affected by AEDs. The Summary of Product Characteristics (SPC) for the Mirena® IUS[10] states that insertion of the device may precipitate a seizure in an epileptic patient because there have been occasional case reports.[7] Women should

Table 22.1

United Kingdom Medical Eligibility Criteria Summary Table Hormonal and Intrauterine Contraception for Women With Epilepsy[9]						
Condition	**Cu-IUD**	**LNG-IUS**	**IMP**	**DMPA**	**POP**	**CHC**
Epilepsy	1	1	1	1	1	1

CHC, Combined hormonal contraception; Cu-IUD, copper intrauterine device; DMPA, depo-medroxyprogesterone acetate; IMP, progestogen-only implant; LNG-IUS, levonorgestrel-releasing intrauterine system; POP, progestogen-only pill. Reproduced under licence from FSRH. Copyright ©Faculty of Sexual and Reproductive Healthcare 2006 to 2016.

be reassured that this is rare and counselled that intrauterine methods may well be their optimal choice, especially if on teratogenic AEDs or EIAEDs. It is often appropriate to refer a woman with epilepsy to a specialist sexual and reproductive healthcare service for intrauterine contraceptive device insertion. Women and girls with epilepsy will need thorough counselling throughout their reproductive life, particularly when changes to their treatment are being considered, to facilitate optimal contraception decision-making.

Table 22.2 summarises the benefits and risks associated with different methods for women with epilepsy.

Table 22.2

Benefits and Risks of Contraceptive Methods		
Type	**Benefits**	**Risks and Disadvantages**
Cu-intrauterine device (Cu-IUD)	• Highly effective for 5 or 10 years • Not affected by antiepileptic drugs (AEDs)	• Risk of seizure at the time of insertion (rare)
Intrauterine systems (IUS)	• Highly effective for 3 or 5 years • Not affected by AEDs • Noncontraceptive benefits (e.g., HMB [Mirena® and Levosert®], HRT [Mirena® only])	• Risk of seizure at the time of insertion (rare)
Nexplanon® implant	• Highly effective for 3 years	• Interactions with enzyme-inducing antiepileptic drugs (EIAEDs) (Use condoms in addition and for 28 days after stopping EIAED; avoid if on EIAEDs long term)
Depo-medroxy-progesterone acetate (DMPA) injection	• Highly effective • Not affected by AEDs	• Best avoided if other risk factors for osteoporosis, such as if taking some AEDs (e.g., carbamazepine, phenytoin, primidone, or sodium valproate)
Progestogen-only pill (POP)	• Medium effectiveness as user dependent	• Avoid if taking EIAEDs

Continued

Table 22.2

Benefits and Risks of Contraceptive Methods—cont'd		
Type	**Benefits**	**Risks and Disadvantages**
Combined hormonal contraception (CHC)	• Medium effectiveness as user dependent	• Avoid if taking EIAEDs • If a woman still wishes to continue CHC when taking EIAED, consider use of a minimum 50 mcg (30 mcg + 20 mcg) Ethinylestradiol monophasic pill during treatment and for a further 28 days with a continuous or tricycling regimen plus pill-free interval of 4 days[11]
Emergency contraception (EC)	• Cu-IUD can be used for ongoing contraception • Cu IUD 10 × more effective than oral EC	• The effectiveness of both UPA-EC and LNG-EC could be reduced if a woman is using an EIAED[12] • Double dose (3 mg) of LNG-EC can be used, but effectiveness is unknown. (Use of double-dose UPA-EC is not currently recommended)

EC, Emergency contraception; *EIAED*, Enzyme-inducing antiepileptic drugs; *HMB*, heavy menstrual bleeding; *HRT*, hormone replacement therapy; *LNG-EC*, levonorgestrel emergency contraception; *UPA-EC*, ulipristal acetate emergency contraception.

Anti-epileptic Drugs

The majority of AEDs cross the placenta and are potentially teratogenic with associated increased risks of congenital malformations and foetal growth restriction.[1,2] Women starting and taking these drugs must therefore be aware of their need for the most effective methods of contraception. Women on AEDs should also be counselled with regard to their regimen prepregnancy and changes made if appropriate. If women conceive while taking AEDs, they require early specialist review, as concerns regarding negative effects on the foetus may cause women to abruptly discontinue epilepsy treatment during pregnancy, putting them at risk of seizures.

EIAEDs induce cytochrome P450 (CYP) hepatic enzyme activity and increase the rate of metabolism of oestrogens and progestogens[7] and reduce the efficacy of CHC, progestogen-only pills and the contraceptive implant. Therefore women taking EIAEDs (e.g., carbamazepine, oxcarbazepine, eslicarbazepine, phenytoin, phenobarbital, primidone, rufinamide, felbamate and topiramate) should be counselled about the risk of failure of these contraceptive methods.[5,7] Co-administration of these methods long term with EIAEDs should be avoided, and if used short term, women should use condoms in addition while using the EIAED and for 28 days after stopping the EIAED.[11] The efficacy of intrauterine or injectable methods is not affected by EIAEDs. The SPC for topiramate indicates that this drug induces CYP3A4 enzyme activity in a dose-dependent manner, and that the evidence suggests that low doses do not significantly reduce exposure to contraceptive hormones.[13] However, there is inadequate clinical evidence to assess doses which present a clinically significant effect on pregnancy risk, and therefore Faculty of Sexual & Reproductive Healthcare (FSRH) guidance[11] does not distinguish between low- and high-dose use of topiramate in relation to potential drug interactions with hormonal contraceptives.

If women taking EIAEDs require emergency contraception, they should be offered a copper intrauterine device (Cu-IUD). If a Cu-IUD is unacceptable or unsuitable, a double dose (3 mg) of oral levonorgestrel emergency contraception can be used. Some AEDs are also associated with increased risk of osteoporosis (e.g., long-term use of carbamazepine, phenytoin, primidone or sodium valproate), and for women taking these, depo-medroxyprogesterone acetate (DMPA) is probably best avoided. The majority of non-enzyme-inducing AEDs (e.g., valproate, gabapentin, levetiracetam, tigabine, vigabatrin, zonisamide, ethosuximide, benzodiazepines and pregabalin) do not interact with hormonal contraception.[5,7] Lamotrigine is an exception detailed later.

Sodium valproate

The teratogenicity of sodium valproate has long been identified, and over 10% of exposed children are born with major congenital abnormalities that can be severe and multisystemic.[14] These risks are highest when valproate is used in high doses and as part of polytherapy with other AEDs.[2,6] Exposed children are also seven times more likely to have developmental delay and five times more likely to have autism spectrum disorder.[14] In April 2018, the Medicines and Healthcare Products Regulatory Agency issued strengthened guidance on valproate because of high rates of congenital malformations and developmental abnormalities. This states that valproate must not be used in pregnancy, and only used in girls and women when there is no alternative and a pregnancy prevention plan is in place.[15] Valproate does not interact with, or affect the efficacy of, any contraceptive method. Valproate may also induce polycystic ovary syndrome with associated hyperandrogenism, menstrual disturbances and anovulatory cycles, which may also affect contraception choice. The underlying mechanisms are not completely understood but thought to involve an interaction with sex steroid synthesis and metabolism in the ovary.[8]

Lamotrigine

Lamotrigine, although not an enzyme-inducing drug, has important interactions with CHC. CHC increases the metabolism of lamotrigine, most likely by increased glucuronidation, and reduces serum levels of lamotrigine.[7] This can lead to decreased seizure control in the active hormone phase. Conversely, increased lamotrigine exposure in the hormone-free week can increase risk of toxicity, with associated side effects of dizziness, ataxia and diplopia.[11,16] Risks of using CHC alongside lamotrigine may thus outweigh the benefits, and current FSRH guidance recommends alternative methods be considered.[11] Desogestrel might increase lamotrigine levels and adverse effects, although there is limited data on this.[16] There is no interaction between long-acting forms of progestogen-only contraceptives (implants, injections and the levonorgestrel-containing intrauterine system) and lamotrigine, and contraceptive efficacy is unaffected.[16] Lamotrigine is generally thought to be the safest AED for use in pregnancy, so women with well-controlled epilepsy on other AEDs may be changed onto this drug before conception. Specialist monitoring is required and dose adjustment may be required in the third trimester.[2]

KEY POINTS

- Unplanned pregnancy in women with epilepsy carries additional risks to mother and child

- Women with epilepsy should be given effective contraception, timely preconception counselling and specialist care to ensure that pregnancy occurs during good seizure control and optimal maternal health

- Women with epilepsy should be counselled as to the risks and benefits of different drug treatments, contraceptive methods and potential interactions

- Women and girls started on teratogenic antiepileptic drugs require a pregnancy prevention plan, and sodium valproate should only be used when alternative treatments are not suitable

- For women on enzyme-inducing antiepileptic drugs and teratogenic drugs, the most effective long-acting reversible contraception methods should be recommended, and intrauterine methods are often optimal

References

1. Nelson-Piercy C. Neurological problems. In: Handbook of obstetric medicine. 5th ed. London: CRC Press; 2015.
2. Bhatia M, Adcock JE, Mackillop L. The management of pregnant women with epilepsy: a multidisciplinary collaborative approach to care. Obstet Gynaecol 2017;19:279–288.
3. Knight M, Kenyon S, Brocklehurst P, Neilson J, Shakespeare J, Kurinczuk J, on behalf of MBRACE-UK. Saving Lives, Improving Mother's Care – Lessons Learned to Inform Future Maternity Care from the UK and Ireland Confidential Enquiries into Maternal Deaths and Morbidity 2009–2012. Oxford: National Perinatal Epidemiology Unit, University of Oxford; 2014.
4. Viale L, Allotey J, Cheong-See F, et al. Epilepsy in pregnancy and reproductive outcomes: a systematic review and meta-analysis. Lancet 2015;386: 1845-1852.
5. RCOG. Epilepsy in Pregnancy (Green-top Guideline No. 68). London, UK: Royal College of Obstetricians and Gynaecologists 2016.
6. National Institute for Health and Care Excellence. Epilepsies: diagnosis and management (NICE) CG137. 2016. https://www.nice.org.uk/guidance/cg137.
7. Marsh M, Kumar U (2008) Practical recommendations for contraception. In: Panayiotopoulos CP, Crawford PM, Thomson T (eds) Educational kit on epilepsies, vol 4. Epilepsy and women. Medicinae, Oxford, pp 96–104
8. Reimers A. Contraception for women with epilepsy: counseling, choices, and concerns. Open Access J Contracept 2016;7:69–76.
9. Faculty of Sexual & Reproductive Healthcare. UK medical eligibility criteria for contraceptive use. 2016. https://www.fsrh.org/standards-and-guidance/external/ukmec-2016-digital- version/.
10. Revised SPC: Mirena (levonorgestrel) 20 micrograms/24 hours intrauterine delivery system. Electronic Medicines Compendium – eMC. 28 May 2020. https://www.medicines.org.uk/emc/product/1132/smpc (Accessed 28 March 2021).
11. Faculty of Sexual & Reproductive Healthcare. Drug interactions with hormonal contraception. 2017. https://www.fsrh.org/documents/ceu-clinical-guidance-drug-interactions-with-hormonal/.
12. Faculty of Sexual & Reproductive Healthcare. Emergency contraception. 2017. https://www.fsrh.org/standards-and-guidance/current-clinical-guidance/emergency-contraception/.
13. SPC: Topamax 25 mg Tablets. Electronic Medicines Compendium – eMC. 25 January 2021. https://www.medicines.org.uk/emc/product/1442/smpc (Accessed 28 March 2021).
14. Wieck A, Jones S. Dangers of valproate in pregnancy. BMJ 2018;361:k1609.

15. Press release: Valproate banned without the pregnancy prevention programme. Medicines and Healthcare products Regulatory Agency; 24 April, 2018. https://www.gov.uk/government/news/valproate-banned-without-the-pregnancy-prevention-programme
16. Stockley's Drug Interactions. Progestogen-only contraception + Lamotrigine. Medicines Complete. 2019. https://www.medicinescomplete.com/#/content/stockley/x12-4633

Emergency Contraception

SHRUTI BATHAM • USHA KUMAR

Case

Toni, 32 years of age, visits the sexual health clinic on Monday requesting emergency contraception (EC). She has been using combined oral contraceptive pills (COCP) for the last 4 years. She has a 5-year-old child and subsequently has had an ectopic pregnancy and two surgical terminations of pregnancy (STOP), with the last STOP only 2 months ago. Her last three pregnancies were unplanned and had resulted from contraceptive pill failure because of missed pills. She has had the same partner for many years, and her recent sexually transmitted infection (STI) screen was clear. She is up to date with her cervical smears. A medical history of note being migraine without aura for many years which has not worsened on COCP. She is not on any other prescription or over-the-counter medication, including St John's wort. There is no contraindication in her family history for using COCP.

Toni has a body mass index (BMI) of 31 kg/m^2 and smokes 10 cigarettes/day. She restarted the COCP immediately after STOP and has not missed pills for the last 2 months. She has always taken the COCP in the traditional way, that is, 21 days of pills followed by 7 days of break.

Her 7-day hormone-free interval (HFI) should have ended on Friday last week and she was supposed to start her new pack of pills on Saturday. However, having visited her friend over the weekend, she forgot her pills and had unprotected sexual intercourse (UPSI) with her partner on Sunday. She took her COCP when back home on Monday and rushed to the clinic for EC because she was worried that she was 2 days late starting her new pill packet and wanted to avoid another unplanned pregnancy.

She is aware of copper coil being the most effective method of EC but considers it invasive and preferred to take oral EC pills. She wants to continue on COCP after EC, with a reminder on phone going forward.

Management

Toni has extended her HFI to 9 days by not taking her COCP on time. Essentially, she has missed two pills in the first week of her pill packet and started the pill on day 10. Because earliest ovulation can occur as early as day 8 of HFI, UPSI on day 9 could expose her to a risk of pregnancy; hence she needs EC.

She was asked about any other UPSI in the HFI to identify which hormonal EC would be suitable for her. She clarified that she did have UPSI with her partner on Thursday morning last week.

She wants to have the best oral EC pill because does not want to risk pregnancy. Levonelle® (Levonorgestrel/LNG-EC) will not work because her first UPSI was about 100 hours ago on Thursday morning. She has heard that ellaOne (Ulipristal acetate/UPA-EC) is a more effective pill. Although UPA-EC pill covers UPSI within the previous 120 hours, in this case, because of the COCP taken on Monday, there is circulating progestogen, which could make UPA potentially less effective.

Although she is not keen on intrauterine device (IUD), it remains her only EC choice as she is within 120 hours from her first UPSI in the HFI. Earliest implantation is believed to occur 6 days after ovulation, which will be on day 14 of an extended HFI. Hence, an IUD can be fitted up to day 13 of the extended HFI, before implantation of a fertilized egg, and will cover multiple episodes of UPSI during this period.

This was explained to Tony, alongside other benefits of the IUD, such as high reliability as an EC option and also providing an effective long-acting reversible form of contraception which will become immediately effective after insertion. Toni accepted IUD for EC and also agreed that the IUD would be a better method for her long-term contraception because she has been forgetful with COCP previously. There are also other factors in her history like smoking, migraine and being obese, which could increase her cardiovascular risks with COCP.

She was counselled about the mode of action, efficacy, duration of use, possible changes to menstrual periods (intermenstrual bleeding, heavier, painful and prolonged periods), expulsion (one in 20 risk), small risk of infection, IUD insertion procedure, including analgesia and the small risk of perforation (up to 2 per 1000 insertions). She was reassured that her overall risk of ectopic pregnancy when using an IUD would be very low. However, in the rare event of an IUD failure, as there could be an increased risk of ectopic pregnancy, she was advised to seek medical advice if she ever missed a period or had abnormal vaginal bleeding or abdominal pain. She consented to have an IUD insertion. A T-Safe copper 380 IUD with a 10-year license was inserted in clinic the same day and she tolerated the procedure well. She was taught how to self-check for the threads and to report if nonpalpable threads or can feel the stem of the IUD. She was also advised to report if she develops any symptoms of pelvic infection. A follow-up was arranged to have a urine pregnancy test after 21 days along with her IUD check.

Introduction

EC is recommended if there is a potential risk of pregnancy after UPSI and the women does not wish to conceive. EC is meant for occasional use only and does not replace regular contraception.[1]

There are specific time frames after UPSI within which EC needs to be initiated for it to be effective and this varies with the different types of EC options available. EC methods work by either disrupting ovulation, preventing fertilization or implantation; they do not disrupt an already implanted pregnancy; thus, EC does not cause abortion.[1]

Prerequisite for emergency contraception

The clinician needs to establish:[2]

1. Likelihood of pregnancy risk from UPSI
2. If already pregnant from any previous UPSI
3. Likelihood of UPSI after EC

Likelihood of pregnancy risk

There are many factors affecting the probability of pregnancy, like the timing of UPSI in relation to the fertile period in a woman's menstrual cycle, age, fertility of the couple, contraception used incorrectly or not used and so on. Sperm can survive up to 5 days after UPSI in upper genital tract, whereas an ovum will survive for less than 24 hours. Risk of pregnancy is highest after UPSI that takes place during the 6 days leading up to and including the day of ovulation.[1]

Ovulation occurs about 14 days before onset of menstruation. One can estimate the earliest ovulation day by taking 14 days away from the 'shortest cycle' length. For example, for 28-day cycle, earliest ovulation is day 14, and fertile window would be between days 9 and 14. The risk of pregnancy is highest during this fertile period with a single episode of UPSI resulting in pregnancy in about 30% of cases.[2,3] However, prediction of fertile period is only applicable if the cycle is regular with last menstrual period (LMP) accurately known.[3] The fertile period can vary between women and also in different cycles for a woman making it difficult to estimate.

It is possible for a woman to get pregnant following UPSI on most days of her natural menstrual cycle; however, there is negligible probability of pregnancy in the first 3 days.[1,2]

Implanted pregnancy risk

If a woman requiring oral EC for UPSI in the last 5 days has also had UPSI more than 21 days ago and has not had a normal menstrual period since the earlier UPSI, a high-sensitivity urine pregnancy test should be done before oral EC is taken. It is worth noting that a negative pregnancy test may not reliably exclude pregnancy if there has been UPSI fewer than 21 days previously and the test needs to be repeated after the 3 week window period.

The clinician needs to establish the woman's LMP and if it was lighter/heavier, shorter or later than normal, as these may indicate pregnancy. One may need to also check on recent delivery, breastfeeding or taken EC as these cause period irregularities.[2]

Unprotected sexual intercourse after emergency contraception

The clinician should also ensure that a discussion about ongoing contraception has taken place in any EC consultation to prevent future pregnancy risk. This is important for oral EC methods because they delay ovulation, and hence there is a risk of pregnancy from subsequent UPSI in the same cycle.[1,2]

Methods of emergency contraception

There are two methods of EC: copper intrauterine device (Cu-IUD) and oral EC. The oral methods include UPA and LNG. Cu-IUD is 10 times more effective EC than oral EC methods and provides immediately effective ongoing contraception.[4]

Table 23.1 details EC methods available in the United Kingdom and their indications as per the Faculty of Sexual & Reproductive Healthcare (FSRH) guidelines.[1]

Table 23.1

Emergency Contraception Methods in the United Kingdom			
Method	**Class**	**Recommended dose/use**	**Indications**
Cu-IUD (copper intrauterine device)	Intrauterine contraceptive method	IUD retained until pregnancy excluded (e.g., onset of next menstrual period) or kept for ongoing contraception	Within 5 days (120 hours) after the first unprotected sexual intercourse (UPSI) in a cycle or within 5 days after the earliest estimated date of ovulation
LNG-EC (Levonorgestrel emergency contraception)	Progestogen	1.5 mg single oral dose[a]	Licensed for use within 72 hours after UPSI or contraceptive failure
UPA-EC (Ulipristal acetate emergency contraception)	Progesterone receptor modulator	30 mg single oral dose	Licensed for use within 5 days (120 hours) after UPSI or contraceptive failure

[a]A double dose (3 mg) of LNG-EC is recommended if a woman is taking an enzyme-inducing drug or if she has a body mass index >26 kg/m^2 or weight >70 kg. Reproduced under licence from FSRH. Copyright © Faculty of Sexual and Reproductive Healthcare December 2017.

The effectiveness of the EC methods are summarized in Table 23.2.[1]

Table 23.2

Effectiveness of Emergency Contraception Methods		
Cu-IUD	**UPA-EC**	**LNG-EC**
Most effective	More effective than LNG-EC.[5] Consider as first-line oral emergency contraception (EC) when unprotected sexual intercourse (UPSI) is likely to have taken place during the 5 days before the estimated day of ovulation, when the risk of pregnancy is highest. Only oral EC that is likely to be effective if UPSI took place 96–120 hours ago	Ineffective if taken more than 96 hours after UPSI

Continued

Table 23.2

Effectiveness of Emergency Contraception Methods—cont'd		
Cu-IUD	**UPA-EC**	**LNG-EC**
Overall pregnancy rate <0.1%	Overall pregnancy rate 1%–2% when taken within 120 hours of UPSI	Overall pregnancy rate 0.6%–2.6% when taken within 72 hours of UPSI
Effective after ovulation	Ineffective after ovulation	Ineffective after ovulation
No decline in efficacy with time since UPSI	No decline in efficacy with time since UPSI (≤120 hours)[5]	Efficacy declines with time after UPSI so needs to be taken as soon as possible

Indications for emergency contraception

EC is indicated if a woman desires to prevent a pregnancy following UPSI in the following scenarios:

1. Not on any contraception
2. Failure of barrier method, such as burst/slipped condom, dislodged cap/diaphragm
3. Potential failure of hormonal/intrauterine contraception
4. Sexual assault
5. After pregnancy:
   - UPSI from day 21 after childbirth unless all criteria for lactational amenorrhoea method are met
   - UPSI from day 5 after miscarriage, abortion, ectopic pregnancy or uterine evacuation for gestational trophoblastic disease

Table 23.3[1] from FSRH guidelines gives a detailed overview on EC management when hormonal/intrauterine contraception has been compromised.

Table 23.3

Emergency Contraception Management when Hormonal/ Intrauterine Contraception has been Compromised		
Method	**Situation leading to possible contraceptive failure**	**Indication for Emergency Contraception**
Hormonal methods	Failure to use additional contraceptive precautions when starting the method	Unprotected sexual intercourse (UPSI) or barrier failure during time that additional precautions required
Combined hormonal transdermal patch/ vaginal ring	Patch detachment or ring removal for >48 hours	If patch detachment or ring removal occurs in week 1 and there has been UPSI or barrier failure during the hormone-free interval (HFI) or week 1
	Extension of patch/ ring free interval by >48 hours	If the HFI is extended, Cu-IUD (copper intrauterine device) can be offered up to 13 days after the start of the HFI assuming previous perfect use
		If CHC has been used in the 7 days before emergency contraception (EC), the effectiveness of UPA-EC could be reduced. Consider LNG-EC
Combined oral contraceptive pill (COCP) (monophasic pill containing ethinylestradiol)	Missed pills: two or more active pills are missed	If the pills are missed in week 1 and there has been UPSI or barrier failure during the pill-free interval or week 1.
		If HFI is extended, Cu-IUD can be offered up to 13 days after the start of the HFI assuming previous perfect use
		If COC has been taken in the 7 days before EC, UPA-EC effectiveness could be reduced. Consider LNG-EC
Combined hormonal contraception (CHC), progestogen-only pill and progestogen-only implant	Failure to use additional contraceptive precautions whilst using liver enzyme inducing drugs or in the 28 days after use	If UPSI or barrier failure during, or in the 28 days following, use of liver enzyme-inducing drugs. Offer a Cu-IUD or LNG-EC double dose. UPA-EC not recommended

Continued

Table 23.3

Emergency Contraception Management when Hormonal/Intrauterine Contraception has been Compromised—cont'd		
Method	**Situation leading to possible contraceptive failure**	**Indication for Emergency Contraception**
Progestogen only pill (POP)	Late or missed pill >27 hours since last traditional POP or >36 hours since last desogestrel-only pill	If a pill is late or missed and UPSI or barrier failure before efficacy has been reestablished (i.e., 48 hours after restarting) Timing of ovulation after missed pills cannot be accurately predicted Cu-IUD is recommended up to 5 days after the first UPSI following a missed POP If POP has been taken in the 7 days before EC, UPA-EC effectiveness could be reduced. Consider LNG-EC
Progestogen only injectable	Late injection (>14 weeks since last injection of Depo-medroxyprogesterone acetate [DMPA])	If there has been UPSI or barrier failure more than 14 weeks after the last injection or within the first 7 days after late injection Timing of ovulation after expiry of the progestogen only injectable is extremely variable Cu-IUD is only recommended up to 5 days after the first UPSI that takes place > 14 weeks after the last DMPA injection. UPA-EC effectiveness could be reduced by residual circulating progestogen. Consider LNG-EC
Progestogen only implant	Expired implant	Progestogen-only implant has exceeded its recommended duration of use and UPSI UPA-EC effectiveness in the presence of progestogen from a recently expired implant is unknown. Consider LNG-EC with immediate appropriate quick start of HC

Table 23.3

	Situation leading to possible contraceptive failure	Indication for Emergency Contraception
Emergency Contraception Management when Hormonal/ Intrauterine Contraception has been Compromised—cont'd		
Method		
Intrauterine contraception (Cu-IUD and LNG-IUS)	Removal without immediate replacement; partial or complete expulsion; threads missing and IUD location unknown	If UPSI has taken place in the 7 days before removal, perforation, partial or complete expulsion Oral EC indicated if UPSI in the last 5 days Depending on the timing of UPSI and time since IUD known to be correctly placed, it may be appropriate to fit another Cu-IUD for EC

Reproduced under licence from FSRH. Copyright © Faculty of Sexual and Reproductive Healthcare December 2017.

How emergency contraception works

Table 23.4 describes how the various type of EC work, advantages, disadvantages and factors which can affect their effectiveness.[1]

Table 23.4

Emergency Contraception: Mode of Action, Advantages, Disadvantages and Factors Affecting Effectiveness

	Cu-IUD	UPA-EC	LNG-EC
Primary mechanism of action	Inhibition of fertilisation by its toxic effect on sperm and ova Copper adversely effects motility and viability of sperm and viability and transport of ova	Inhibiting or delaying ovulation for at least 5 days Delays ovulation even if given after onset of luteinising hormone (LH) surge, but before the peak	Inhibiting or delaying ovulation for 5 days, if taken before LH surge Not effective if given after the onset of LH surge

Continued

Table 23.4

Emergency Contraception: Mode of Action, Advantages, Disadvantages and Factors Affecting Effectiveness—cont'd			
	Cu-IUD	**UPA-EC**	**LNG-EC**
Other mechanism of action	Local endometrial inflammatory reaction prevents implantation	No effect on endometrial receptivity or implantation	No effect on endometrial receptivity or implantation
Advantages	Only method of emergency contraception (EC) that is effective after ovulation Effective both pre- and post-fertilisation Immediately effective ongoing contraception	More effective than LNG-EC Effective up to 120 hours after unprotected sexual intercourse (UPSI)	Hormonal contraception (HC) can be immediately started after LNG-EC with additional precautions till HC becomes effective
Disadvantages	Invasive procedure Pain associated with procedure Expulsion (1 in 20 risk) Intrauterine device (IUD) displacement Perforation (≤2 per 1000 insertions)	Cannot inhibit ovulation at or after LH peak Does not provide ongoing contraception Need to wait for 5 days before starting HC after UPA-EC with additional precautions till HC becomes effective	Cannot work if LH surge has started Does not provide ongoing contraception
Factors affecting effectiveness of method			
Body mass index (BMI)/ weight	Unaffected	Potentially less effective if weight >85 kg or BMI >30 kg/m^2 • Double dose not recommended	Reduced effectiveness with BMI >26 kg/m^2 or weight >70kg • Double dose an option – effectiveness not known

Table 23.4

Emergency Contraception: Mode of Action, Advantages, Disadvantages and Factors Affecting Effectiveness—cont'd

	Cu-IUD	UPA-EC	LNG-EC
Post bariatric surgery and malabsorption conditions, (e.g., Crohn disease)	Unaffected	Reduced because of malabsorption	Reduced because of malabsorption
Drugs inducing diarrhoea and/or vomiting, (e.g., Orlistat, laxatives)	Unaffected	Reduced	Reduced

Drug interactions[a]

	Cu-IUD	UPA-EC	LNG-EC
Hepatic enzyme (CYP450) inducing drugs	Unaffected	Reduced during and for 28 days after use of drugs; Double dose not recommended	Reduced during and for 28 days after use of drugs; Double dose an option – effectiveness not known
Gastric pH increasing drugs	None	Caution required, although unknown clinical significance	None
Progestogen containing drugs[b]	None	Effectiveness reduced if progestogen containing drugs taken within 5 days after taking UPA[6,7] or during the 7 days before UPA-EC	None

[a]Refer to BNF[8] for the full list of interacting medicines with oral EC
[b]Progestogen containing drugs include combined hormonal contraception (CHC), progestogen only pills (POP), subdermal Implant (SDI), depo-medroxyprogesterone acetate (DMPA), levonorgestrel intrauterine system (LNG-IUS), hormone replacement therapy (HRT)[1]

It is to be noted that the currently recommended human immunodeficiency virus (HIV) post-exposure prophylaxis by British Association for Sexual Health and HIV (BASHH), Truvada (tenofovir and emtricitabine) and Raltegravir, are not liver enzyme inducing drugs and do not lower efficacy of oral EC.[1]

Special considerations

Copper intrauterine device

No contraception and regular cycle. A pregnancy does not implant during the first 5 days after fertilisation, and earliest implantation is only at 6 days after ovulation. Cu-IUD can be fitted in this time, that is, up to 5 days after the first UPSI or 5 days after the earliest likely ovulation, whichever is the later. For example, for a 28-day cycle, it can be fitted up to day 19, irrespective of the number of UPSI earlier in the cycle.[1,2]

Not using hormonal contraception and amenorrhoeic. Cu-IUD can be given to a woman who is amenorrhoeic if all recent UPSI have occurred in last 5 days, no other UPSI in last 21 days and highly sensitive urine pregnancy test (HSUPT) is negative. HSUPT detects human chorionic gonadotropin levels around 20 mIU/mL.[1]

Hormonal contraception compromised: combined hormonal contraception. A systematic review reported earliest ovulation at 8 days after the last correctly taken pill in previous pill packet.[9] Because the earliest implantation is only at 6 days after ovulation, Cu-IUD can be inserted up to 13 days after start of the HFI, provided the CHC was used correctly before HFI; this ensures that CU-IUD is inserted before implantation.[1]

Hormonal contraception compromised: progestogen-only implant. Cu-IUD insertion for EC- after recently removed implant.
Because ovulation returns rapidly after removal of an implant, a Cu-IUD can be inserted up to 5 days after first UPSI following implant removal.[1]

Oral emergency contraception

Use of oral emergency contraception if there has also been unprotected sexual intercourse earlier in the cycle. There is no evidence that UPA or LNG-EC disrupt existing pregnancy or negatively affect pregnancy outcomes if taken in very early pregnancy.[10,11] Based on this safety data, if a woman has had UPSI earlier in the cycle (more than 5 days before presenting for EC, as well as within the last 5 days) and could be at risk of very early pregnancy, UPA-EC can still be used.[1]

Similarly, LNG-EC can be used if there has been UPSI earlier in the cycle, as well as within the last 4 days.[1]

Use of oral emergency contraception more than once in a cycle. Because LNG and UPA-EC work by delaying ovulation, there could be a three- to four fold increase in risk of pregnancy from further acts of UPSI, compared with no UPSI in the same cycle.[12] Based on the half-life of LNG and UPA, repeat use of EC is recommended in the case of further UPSI beyond 24 hours from the last EC use.[13]

Oral EC can be used more than once in a cycle as per the following directions:[1]

1. If already taken UPA-EC once or more in a cycle, UPA-EC can be offered again after further UPSI in the same cycle
2. If already taken UPA-EC, LNG-EC should not be taken in the following 5 days
3. If already taken LNG-EC once or more in a cycle, LNG-EC can be offered again after further UPSI in the same cycle
4. If already taken LNG-EC, UPA-EC could be less effective if taken in following 7 days

Contraindications/restrictions

EC is generally considered safe for most patients.

Copper intrauterine device

Contraindications for Cu-IUD as EC are the same as those for routine IUD insertion. Because of the potential risk of ascending pelvic infection associated with insertion of an IUD in women with existing bacterial STI, such as *Chlamydia trachomatis* or *Neisseria gonorrhoea*, all women requesting insertion of IUC should be individually assessed regarding risk of STI and STI screening carried out where indicated.[1,14,15]

Antibiotic prophylaxis may be considered for women who require an emergency IUD insertion if there is significant risk of STI.[14]

If a woman has asymptomatic chlamydia infection, Cu-IUD insertion for EC may be considered after discussion of the risks and benefits with the patient and with appropriate antibiotic cover. However, if she has symptomatic chlamydia or current *N. gonorrhoea* infection, then antibiotic treatment should be completed before insertion of a Cu-IUD.[1]

Previous ectopic pregnancy, young age and nulliparity are not contraindications to IUD use.[15]

Oral emergency contraception

UK medical eligibility criteria (UKMEC) 2016[15] includes no contra-indications to the use of LNG or UPA-EC. Thus women can be reassured that oral EC for occasional use is safe.

Table 23.5 highlights specific medical conditions where there are no restrictions or where benefits outweigh risks for use of EC according to UKMEC.[15]

Table 23.5

Specific Medical Conditions		
Clinical condition	**UPA-EC**	**LNG-EC**
Severe hepatic impairment	UK medical eligibility criteria (UKMEC) category 1	UKMEC category 1
Acute intermittent porphyria	UKMEC category 2[a]	UKMEC category 2[a]
Breast cancer	UPA-EC Category 2[b]	UKMEC Category 2[b]

[a]Acute attacks may be precipitated by oestrogens and progestogens and 1% can be fatal; women may use UPA or LNG following discussion of the risks and benefits and with clinical judgement.
[b]Although the prognosis of women with breast cancer may be affected by hormonal contraception, the benefit of oral emergency contraception is considered to outweigh the risk.[15]

Restrictions/caution advised. Table 23.6 shows restriction/caution advised by Summary of Product Characteristics (SPC) for ellaOne and Levonelle®.[16,17]

Table 23.6

Restrictions/Caution		
Clinical condition	**UPA-EC**	**LNG-EC**
Severe asthma controlled by oral glucocorticoids[a]	Avoid	
Galactose intolerance and lapp lactase deficiency and glucose-galactose malabsorption	Avoid; contains lactose	Avoid; contains lactose
Hypersensitivity	Avoid if hypersensitivity to UPA	Avoid if hypersensitivity to LNG

[a]SPC for ellaOne advises against use in women with severe asthma controlled with oral steroids because of the antiglucocorticoid effect of UPA.

Breast feeding and emergency contraception[1]

Table 23.7 shows advice with regards to EC and breast feeding.

Table 23.7

Emergency Contraception and Breastfeeding		
CU-IUD	**UPA-EC**	**LNG-EC**
Higher relative risk of perforation during intrauterine device insertion in the postpartum period and during breastfeeding. Absolute risk still low (about 6/1000 within 36 weeks of delivery)[18] UK medical eligibility criteria category 3 between 48 hours and 28 days of delivery because of increased perforation and expulsion risk[15]	Advised not to breastfeed and to express and discard milk for a week after taking UPA-EC[a]	No adverse effects on lactation or on the infant

[a]Safety of UPA-EC during breast feeding has not been studied.

Side effects of emergency contraception[1,14,16,17]

Table 23.8 summarises the side effects of EC.

Table 23.8

Side Effects of Emergency Contraception			
Side effects	**Cu-IUD**	**UPA-EC**	**LNG-EC**
Dysmenorrhoea	✓	✓(10% of users)	✓(10% of users)
Headache, nausea		✓(10% of users)	✓(10% of users)
Menstrual disturbances	Heavier Periods	75%: next period at expected time or within 7 days of expected time 20%: next period more than 7 days late 4%: next period more than 20 days late 10%: intermenstrual bleeding	Majority of women menstruate within 7 days of expected time after LNG-EC Fewer than 10% have it delayed by 7 days

If vomiting occurs within 3 hours of taking oral EC, a repeat dose should be given.[1]

Pregnancy outcome following failed emergency contraception

There is no evidence of adverse pregnancy outcomes or foetal abnormalities after exposure to LNG or UPA EC.[10,11]

There does not appear to be an increased risk of ectopic pregnancy following use of Cu-IUD[4] as EC, UPA[11] or LNG.[19]

The overall risk of ectopic pregnancy is reduced with use of IUC when compared with using no contraception. However, if a pregnancy does occur with an intrauterine method in situ, the risk of an ectopic pregnancy occurring is increased; IUC users should be informed about symptoms of ectopic pregnancy and advised to seek medical assessment.[14]

Future contraception after oral emergency contraception

The clinician should find details of contraception previously used and any problems associated with that method as it would influence future contraception method.[1]

A full choice of contraception should be offered and discussed after checking eligibility criteria.[15]

After LNG-EC women can immediately quick start suitable hormonal contraception, such as CHC (except cyproterone acetate containing COC), POP, implant and perform a urine pregnancy test 21 days later to exclude pregnancy from EC failure. DMPA is only considered for quick start if other methods are declined. They must be advised to use condoms reliably or abstain from sex until contraception becomes effective (7 days for CHC, 9 days for Qlaira, 7 days for implant and DMPA, 2 days for POP). If an intrauterine hormonal contraception (IUS) is chosen, insertion will need to be deferred until after a pregnancy is excluded.[20]

After taking UPA-EC, commencement of CHC, POP, Implant and DMPA should be delayed for 5 days (at least 120 hours), as immediate quick starting of hormonal contraception after UPA could potentially impair the ability of UPA-EC to delay ovulation and reduce its effectiveness.[1,6,7] They must use condoms reliably or abstain from sex during the 5 days waiting and then until their contraceptive method is effective. However, there is one specific exception to this. In established COC pill users on a 21/7 regimen, if after the pill-free interval, in the first week, they restart the pill for 4 days and subsequently miss the next 3 consecutive pills, UPA-EC may be offered with immediate restart of COC and condom use for

7 days.[21] This is based on a recent study which has shown that in the above specific scenario, ovulation and theoretical risk of pregnancy later in the cycle was less likely when COC was restarted immediately after UPA-EC than if COC restart was delayed for 5 days after UPA-EC.[22]

Follow-up after emergency contraception

A urine pregnancy test is advised if after EC the next menstrual period is delayed by more than 7 days, or is unusually lighter or is associated with abdominal pain.

Women who quickly start hormonal contraception after EC should have a urine pregnancy test 21 days from the last UPSI irrespective of whether they have a bleed, as bleeding associated with the contraceptive method may not represent a menstrual bleed.

KEY POINTS

- There are two methods of emergency contraception (EC): Cu-IUD (copper intrauterine device) and oral EC. Oral EC include UPA-EC and LNG-EC.

- LNG-EC is licensed for use up to 72 hours after unprotected sexual intercourse (UPSI); UPA-EC is licensed for use up to 120 hours after UPSI; a Cu-IUD can be inserted within 120 hours after first UPSI in a cycle or within 5 days after the earliest estimated date of ovulation.

- Cu-IUD is 10 times more effective method than oral methods and must be offered to all women seeking EC unless there are specific contraindications. It also has the advantage of providing immediately effective ongoing contraception. It is not affected by body mass index/weight or by other drugs.

- UPA-EC is more effective than LNG-EC and should be first-line oral EC when UPSI is likely to have taken place during the 5 days before the estimated day of ovulation, when the risk of pregnancy is highest.

- Oral ECs must be taken as soon as possible after UPSI so that it has the best chance of being taken early enough to delay ovulation.

- UPA-EC and LNG-EC are not effective if given after ovulation.

- Efficacy of LNG-EC is reduced in overweight and obese women; For women who weigh over 70 kg or with BMI over 26 kg/m², double dose LNG-EC (3 mg) is required if they decline or are unsuitable for Cu-IUD or UPA-EC.

- Efficacy of LNG-EC and UPA-EC is reduced during and for 28 days after use of liver enzyme inducing medication. If Cu-IUD declined, double dose LNG-EC (3 mg) could be considered off-licence.

- Efficacy of UPA-EC could be affected by progestogen containing medications taken during the previous 7 days and the following 5 days.

- Both UPA-EC and LNG-EC can be given more than once in a cycle and do not disrupt an ongoing pregnancy.

- Oral EC do not provide ongoing contraception. There is a risk of pregnancy from UPSI following oral EC because of delayed ovulation. Hence, it is essential that after oral EC women commence ongoing reliable contraception.

- Following LNG-EC a woman can quick start ongoing contraception immediately, whereas after UPA-EC, quick start hormonal contraception needs to be delayed by 5 days.

- Sexually transmitted infection risk assessment is an essential part of any consultation where there has been UPSI.

- Choosing the right EC: Refer Appendix A and B for the Faculty of Sexual & Reproductive Healthcare algorithms.[1]

Appendix A: Decision-making Algorithms for Emergency Contraception[1]

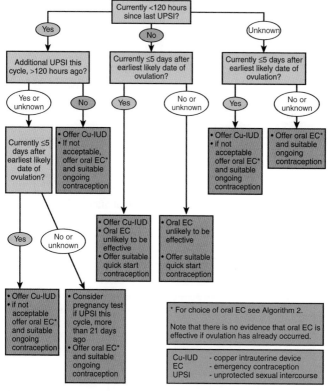

Reproduced under licence from FSRH. Copyright © Faculty of Sexual and Reproductive Healthcare 2017.

Appendix B: Decision-Making Algorithm for Oral Emergency Contraception (EC): Levonorgestrel EC (LNG-EC) Versus Ulipristal Acetate EC (UPA-EC)[1]

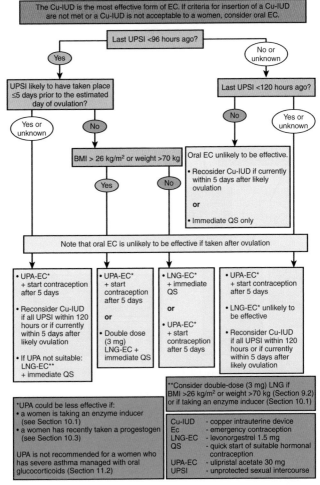

The Cu-IUD is the most effective form of EC. If criteria for insertion of a Cu-IUD are not met or a Cu-IUD is not acceptable to a women, consider oral EC.

Last UPSI <96 hours ago?

Yes → UPSI likely to have taken place ≤5 days prior to the estimated day of ovulation?

No or unknown → Last UPSI <120 hours ago?

UPSI likely to have taken place ≤5 days prior to the estimated day of ovulation?
- Yes or unknown
- No → BMI > 26 kg/m² or weight >70 kg
  - Yes
  - No

Last UPSI <120 hours ago?
- No → Oral EC unlikely to be effective.
  - Reconsider Cu-IUD if currently within 5 days after likely ovulation
  - **or**
  - Immediate QS only
- Yes or unknown

Note that oral EC is unlikely to be effective if taken after ovulation

- UPA-EC*
  + start contraception after 5 days
- Reconsider Cu-IUD if all UPSI within 120 hours or if currently within 5 days after likely ovulation
- If UPA not suitable: LNG-EC**
  + immediate QS

- UPA-EC*
  + start contraception after 5 days
- **or**
- Double dose (3 mg) LNG-EC + immediate QS

- LNG-EC*
  + immediate QS
- **or**
- UPA-EC*
  + start contraception after 5 days

- UPA-EC*
  + start contraception after 5 days
- LNG-EC* unlikely to be effective
- Reconsider Cu-IUD if all UPSI within 120 hours or if currently within 5 days after likely ovulation

---

*UPA could be less effective if:
- a women is taking an enzyme inducer (see Section 10.1)
- a women has recently taken a progestogen (see Section 10.3)

UPA is not recommended for a women who has severe asthma managed with oral glucocorticoids (Section 11.2)

**Consider double-dose (3 mg) LNG if BMI >26 kg/m² or weight >70 kg (Section 9.2) or if taking an enzyme inducer (Section 10.1)

Cu-IUD	- copper intrauterine device
Ec	- emergency contraception
LNG-EC	- levonorgestrel 1.5 mg
QS	- quick start of suitable hormonal contraception
UPA-EC	- ulipristal acetate 30 mg
UPSI	- unprotected sexual intercourse

References

1. FSRH. FSRH Guideline: Emergency Contraception [online]. 2017. <https://www.fsrh.org/standards-and-guidance/documents/ceu-clinical-guidance-emergency-contraception-march-2017/> [accessed 03.04.20].

2. Portal.e-lfh.org.uk. e-SRH 10 - Emergency Contraception [online]. 2012. <https://portal.e-lfh.org.uk/Component/Details/391302> [accessed 30.03.20].

3. Wilcox AJ, Weinberg CR, Baird DD. Timing of sexual intercourse in relation to ovulation. Effects on the probability of conception, survival of the pregnancy, and sex of the baby. N Engl J Med 1995;333:1517–1521.

4. Cleland K, Zhu H, Goldstuck N, Cheng L, Trussell J. The efficacy of intrauterine devices for emergency contraception: a systematic review of 35 years of experience. Hum Reprod 2012;27(7):1994–2000.

5. Glasier AF, Cameron ST, Fine PM, et al. Ulipristal acetate versus levonorgestrel for emergency contraception: a randomised non-inferiority trial and meta-analysis. Lancet 2010;375:555–562.

6. Edelman AB, Jensen JT, McCrimmon S, Messerle-Forbes M, O'Donnell A, Hennebold J. Combined oral contraceptive interference with the ability of ulipristal acetate to delay ovulation: a prospective cohort study. Contraception 2018;98(6)463–466.

7. Brache V, Cochon L, Duijkers IJM, et al. A prospective, randomized, pharmacodynamic study of quick-starting a desogestrel progestin-only pill following ulipristal acetate for emergency contraception. Hum Reprod 2015;30:2785–2793.

8. NICE. Contraceptives, Interactions | Treatment Summary | BNF Content Published By NICE. [online] 2020. Bnf.nice.org.uk. <https://bnf.nice.org.uk/treatment-summary/contraceptives-interactions.html> [accessed 29.03.20].

9. Zapata LB, Steenland MW, Brahmi D, Marchbanks PA, Curtis KM. Effect of missed combined hormonal contraceptives on contraceptive effectiveness: a systematic review. Contraception 2013;87:685–700.

10. Zhang L, Chen J, Wang Y, Ren F, Yu W, Cheng L. Pregnancy outcome after levonorgestrel-only emergency contraception failure: a prospective cohort study. Hum Reprod 2009;24:1605–1611.

11. Levy DP, Jager M, Kapp N, Abitbol JL. Ulipristal acetate for emergency contraception: postmarketing experience after use by more than 1 million women. Contraception 2014;89:431–433.

12. Glasier A, Cameron ST, Blithe D, et al. Can we identify women at risk of pregnancy despite using emergency contraception? Data from randomized trials of ulipristal acetate and levonorgestrel. Contraception 2011;84:363–367.

13. Cameron S, Li H, Gemzell-Danielsson K. Current controversies with oral emergency contraception. BJOG 2017;124(13):1948–1956.

14. FSRH. Intrauterine Contraception. 2015 <https://www.fsrh.org/standards-and-guidance/documents/ceuguidanceintrauterinecontraception/>.

15. FSRH. UK Medical Eligibility Criteria for Contraceptive use [online]. 2016. <https://www.fsrh.org/standards-and-guidance/documents/ukmec-2016/> [accessed 26.03.20].

16. electronic Medicines Compendium (eMC). Bayer PLC. Summary of Product Characteristics: Levonelle 1500 microgram tablet. 20 December 2016. <http://www.medicines.org.uk/emc/medicine/16887>.

17. electronic Medicines Compendium (eMC). HRA Pharma UK and Ireland Limited. Summary of Product Characteristics: ellaOne 30 mg. 22 December 2016. <http://www.medicines.org.uk/emc/medicine/22280>.

18. Heinemann K, Reed S, Moehner S, Minh TD. Risk of uterine perforation with levonorgestrel releasing and copper intrauterine devices in the European Active Surveillance Study on Intrauterine Devices. Contraception 2015;91:274–279.

19. Cleland K, Raymond E, Trussell J, Cheng L, Zhu H. Ectopic pregnancy and emergency contraceptive pills: a systematic review. Obstet Gynecol 2010;115:1263–1266.

20. FSRH. FSRH Guideline: Quick Starting Contraception [online]. 2017. <https://www.fsrh.org/standards-and-guidance/documents/fsrh-clinical-guidance-quick-starting-contraception-april-2017/> [accessed 28.03.20].

21. FSRH, 2020. FSRH CEU Statement: Response to Recent Publication Regarding Banh, et al. [online] Available at: <https://www.fsrh.org/standards-and-guidance/documents/fsrh-ceu-statement-response-to-recent-publication-regarding/>
22. Banh C, Rautenberg T, Duijkers IJ, et al. The effects on ovarian activity of delaying versus immediately restarting combined oral contraception after missing three pills and taking ulipristal acetate 30 mg. Contraception 2020;102(3):145–151.

Contraception and Sexual Health in Transgender Individuals

SHRUTI BATHAM • USHA KUMAR

Case

Tom, a 26-year-old trans male, comes to the sexual health clinic enquiring about emergency contraception (EC). Tom has been told by a friend to go to the sexual health clinic to obtain EC. Tom has been receiving testosterone injection every 4 weeks through the general practitioner (GP) for the last 12 months and is amenorrhoeic, so believes that contraception is not needed.

Tom was first asked for the preferred name and pronoun to be used during consultation. Tom wished to be addressed by name and the pronoun 'they'. Throughout the consultation, gender neutral terminology was used.

Tom was born as female and has gender dysphoria. They are transitioning using gender-affirming hormone therapy to induce characteristics of the desired sex which is male.

Tom has no medical, surgical or mental health history. There is no history of domestic or sexual violence. There is also no relevant family history of note. They are not on any medication except testosterone (Sustanon®) intramuscular injection. GP has been monitoring hormone levels and doing relevant blood tests every 3 months for gender-affirming hormone therapy. Tom is a non-smoker and does not drink alcohol or use recreational drugs. Tom has had regular periods in the past and has only recently engaged in sexual activity. Tom has not had a cervical smear or sexual transmitted infection (STI) screen in the past but has had two doses of human papilloma virus (HPV) vaccination while at school. Their body mass index (BMI) is 25 kg/m^2 and blood pressure (BP) 112/70 mm Hg.

Tom has recently met Harry and had vaginal intercourse without condom 3 days ago, which they found very painful. Harry is a cis male born in the United Kingdom and has had other female partners in the past. His recent STI screen was clear.

Management

Tom was advised that although they have reversible amenorrhoea induced by testosterone, ovarian follicles are not depleted, and hence there is a risk of pregnancy. It was explained that they need EC for unprotected sexual intercourse (UPSI) with a cis male and also an ongoing reliable contraception if they want to avoid pregnancy. It was stressed that testosterone will not affect the efficacy of EC, nor will EC affect testosterone therapy.

EC options available for Tom are intrauterine device (IUD) and oral emergency hormonal contraception (EHC). It was emphasized that IUD is the most effective option, and it will also serve as ongoing method of contraception. Oral EHC includes Levonorgestrel (LNG-EC) and Ulipristal acetate (UPA-EC), with UPA-EC being more effective than LNG-EC.

Oral EHC methods do not provide ongoing contraception, hence they need to start reliable contraception for any further UPSI. Suitable hormonal contraception that could be quick started (QS) after EHC for Tom include oral methods like progestogen-only pills (POP) or long-acting reversible methods (LARC), like subdermal implant (SDI). After LNG-EC, regular hormonal contraception can be QS straightaway, with abstinence from sexual intercourse or use of additional barrier contraception till the method becomes effective. Whereas after UPA-EC, QS of regular hormonal contraceptive method needs to be delayed for 5 days. Additional contraceptive precautions will need to be followed during those 5 days and until regular hormonal contraception becomes effective (2 days for POP and 7 days for SDI).

Depo-Provera® (Depo-Medroxyprogesterone Acetate [DMPA]) is not ideally suited for QS after EHC, unless they deny other reliable contraception. Combined hormonal contraception (CHC) can counteract the masculinising effects of testosterone and will not be suitable to QS in transgender men on testosterone.

Tom was advised they have a risk of acquiring STI because of UPSI and consistent use of condom would reduce STI risk and additionally provide contraception.

Tom was also informed of the need to have STI screen for chlamydia/gonorrhoea (CT/GC) after 2 weeks, human immunodeficiency virus (HIV) screen after 6 weeks and syphilis screen after 3 months from UPSI to cover the incubation period for these infections. They were offered a cervical smear same day and, as they declined, was booked for later.

Tom was offered examination of the internal pelvic area in view of painful intercourse. They were also offered a chaperone, which they declined. Small-size speculum with topical lubricant was used. Vagina showed signs of atrophy, but no ulcers, fissures, oedema or vaginal discharge were noted. It was explained that having painful intercourse could be caused by long-term testosterone treatment causing vaginal atrophy. They were advised to use vaginal oestrogen cream/pessary to help with vaginal dryness because it acts locally and will not interfere with the masculinising effect of testosterone.

Tom declined IUD and opted to take LNG-EC and QS POP. They were advised to abstain from sexual intercourse for next 2 days and do urine pregnancy test after 23 days.

Background

One must remember that gender identity is independent of sexual orientation and should ask open-ended questions when taking a sexual history from transgender individuals. The consultation should always take into account the patient's gender identity and address them by their preferred names and pronouns. Many individuals prefer they/them to he/him or she/her.[1,2]

It may be useful to check/confirm with the patient as to how they wish to refer to their anatomy. There are phrases that are considered to be more gender neutral, such as 'external pelvic area' instead of 'vulva', or 'outer parts' instead of 'labia', and these should be used.[2] All members of clinic staff should be respectful and gender affirming in their behaviour toward the patient.[2]

Some useful terminologies are given here[3]:

Sex: Refers to the sex assigned at birth which is based on genitalia one is born with.

Gender identity: Refers to our inner sense of our gender and relates to the feeling of being a man or woman, both or neither. This is different from Gender Role, which is societal expectation of the way that men and women should behave and express.

Cisgender: Term used to describe a person whose gender identity corresponds with the sex assigned at birth. A *cis man* is one who identifies as a male and was assigned male sex at birth. Similarly, a *cis woman* is one who identifies as a female and was assigned female sex at birth.

Nongender: Relates to situations where some people do not regard themselves as having a gender identity.

Gender dysphoria/variance: Relates to situations where some people experience psychologic discomfort as a result of the conflict between their gender identity and their biologic sex and or/their expected gender role.

Some people may experience extreme discomfort and may wish to change their gender role and their bodies permanently to reflect who they believe they really are. A person may feel compelled to start living full-time in the role that accords with their gender identity, and this is called *transition*.

Transgender (trans) individual is someone whose gender identity is not congruent with the sex they were assigned at birth. *Transgender man* is someone who was born female but identifies as a man. *Transgender woman* is someone who was born male but identifies as a woman. *Nonbinary/gender-queer* describes any gender identity which does not fit the male and female binary.[3]

The World Professional Association for Transgender Health (WPATH) has set out specific clinical guidelines highlighting three stages of gender-affirming interventions with progressive levels of irreversibility.[4] It will be prudent to discuss fertility options, for example, oocyte/sperm cryopreservation, before starting any medical intervention. The guidelines require puberty (Tanner stage 2) to have begun before any intervention is agreed because there may be instances where gender dysphoria may resolve by then.[4,5]

Stage 1: Puberty suppression treatments in which Gonadotrophin-releasing hormone (GnRH) agonists are used.

Stage 2: Gender-affirming hormonal treatment.

Stage 3: Gender-affirming surgery (GAS). See Table 24.1.[2]

Table 24.1[2]

Gender Affirming Surgery (GAS)		
	Trans woman	**Trans man**
Chest Surgery	Breast augmentation	Bilateral mastectomy
		Male chest creation
Genital Surgery	Orchidectomy	Hysterectomy
	Penectomy	Salpingo-oophorectomy
	Vaginoplasty	Vaginectomy
	Vulvoplasty	Metoidoplasty
	Clitoroplasty	Phalloplasty
		Scrotoplasty
		Urethroplasty
		Implantation of penile/ testicular prosthesis
Other Interventions	Phonosurgery	Pectoral Implants
	Facial surgery	Aesthetic surgery
	Gluteal augmentation	
	Aesthetic surgery	

Introduction and epidemiology

Approximately 0.3% to 0.5% of the global population identify as transgender; however, exact prevalence remains unknown.[1] Based on prevalence studies, male-to-female cases outnumber female-to-male cases, with 1 per 10,000 males and 1 per 27,000 females affected by gender dysphoria.[5] The transgender and nonbinary population is increasing, and this is reflected in the number of referrals for transitioning to gender identity clinics (GICs) in the United Kingdom. A GIC offer specialist services to transgender patients, including hormone treatment and GAS. In some cases, GPs may also provide 'bridging prescriptions'.[2]

It is important to understand that many transgender people will need both hormone therapy and surgery to alleviate their gender dysphoria, whereas some require neither.[2] There are unique health needs experienced by transgender individuals especially with regards to their family planning needs.[1]

There are misconceptions regarding fertility and pregnancy risk in the trans community and amongst some clinicians.[1,6,7] For example, trans men on testosterone have amenorrhoea because of testosterone use but are at risk of pregnancy if they are under 55 years of age and not using contraception, not menopausal, have not undergone sterilisation, total abdominal hysterectomy or bilateral salpingo-oophorectomy. Reported rate of contraceptive use among transgender men varies from 20% to 60% according to some studies.[8] Thus unintended pregnancies do occur in this population taking testosterone. In one study, 20% of transgender and gender nonbinary who were assigned female at birth experienced pregnancy while they were amenorrhoeic on testosterone at the time of conception.[8]

Reproductive and sexual health for transgender and nonbinary people

Contraception

Faculty of Sexual & Reproductive Health care (FSRH) Clinical Effectiveness Unit Statement on Contraceptive Choices and Sexual Health for Transgender and Non-Binary People provides guidance on contraceptive choices for transgender and nonbinary people and their partners, who have vaginal sex risking pregnancy.[9]

Contraception counselling involves discussion on what is safe, what does not aggravate gender dysphoria and also what methods will not interfere with the gender affirmation management.[1] The appropriateness and acceptability of different methods of contraception will be determined by the individual's stage of transition. Any advice should include accurate information about the efficacy, risks and side effects, advantages and disadvantages, and noncontraceptive benefits of all available methods.[9]

They need to be informed that condoms provide contraception when used correctly and consistently and also protect against sexually transmitted infections (STIs). The contraceptive failure rate of condoms with perfect (correct and consistent) use is 2% and with typical use failure rate is 13%.[10]

Choices for trans people assigned female at birth

As with any contraceptive counselling, individuals who were female at birth should be given up-to-date accurate information about all methods of contraception and medical eligibility assessed based on personal characteristics, age and any medical conditions or drug therapies.[9] Also when discussing contraceptive options, their future desires for fertility should be taken into account.

Because the process of transitioning is not a uniform one for every individual, besides regular contraceptive history, a check list should include the triggers for gender dysphoria, potential for dysphoria from each contraception method, hormonal affirmation medications being used, surgery done to remove the uterus and/or ovaries and whether the patient is at risk for unwanted pregnancy.[1]

A trans man or nonbinary person who is receiving GnRH analogues to suppress ovarian function or testosterone therapy should be aware that although these can cause amenorrhoea, they do not provide adequate contraceptive cover. Ovulation is impaired but not completely absent. Factors like missed doses, incomplete dosing and switching between testosterone preparations can lead to breakthrough ovulation from incomplete suppression. Also testosterone is a teratogen that is contraindicated in pregnancy. As a result, if pregnancy does occur, then testosterone treatment used in current regimens can be associated with masculinisation of a female foetus, for example, labial fusion, abnormal vaginal development and so on.[8,9]

Transgender population may have additional unique concerns and needs related to factors triggering gender dysphoria. These could be anatomic and/or physiologic like reproductive organs, menstruation etc. Many individuals experience their chest/breast as a significant source of gender dysphoria. Thus hormonal contraceptives (CHC, POP, SDI, DMPA, IUS) that cause chest/breast tenderness may end up exacerbating their dysphoria.[8,11–14] Whereas with oestrogen-containing contraceptives, the tenderness resolves by itself in the first few months, with progestogen only methods, this may persist.[8]

Reversible methods: long-acting reversible contraception (LARC). Transgender men who are unsure of their long-term desires for fertility, should be recommended to use highly effective LARC. Progestin containing LARC such as SDI, DMPA and IUS do not interfere with the hormonal affirmation treatment the individual has been prescribed.[1]

Some individuals may experience dysphoria related to their pelvic anatomy and may prefer to avoid contraception involving pelvic procedures. For patients who accept intrauterine methods but anticipate distress, anxiolytics, local analgesics and placement under sedation can be offered. Smaller IUD and smaller speculum may be useful for those on long-term testosterone with subsequent atrophic changes. A course of vaginal oestrogen before procedure may improve atrophic vaginitis.[8]

There is qualitative evidence indicating that transgender men are interested in suppression of their menstrual cycle and prefer amenorrhoea as this would be more concordant with their transgender identity.[1,8] Progestogen-only injections and the IUS (levonorgestrel intrauterine systems) provide additional noncontraceptive benefit of reducing or stopping vaginal bleeding, which is most often desirable.[9] According to a study on menstrual suppression and contraceptive choices in transgender adolescent and young adults, DMPA was the most commonly used method.[15]

Some trans men do not want to be on testosterone and may just seek menstrual suppression. They should be informed that although DMPA and IUS offer the highest amenorrhoea rates, this is not an immediate effect and may take up to 1 year. Complete amenorrhoea may not happen for everyone.[8]

Irregular bleeding is a side effect of all progestogen only methods and more common with SDI. SDI and DMPA can also very rarely cause breast enlargement.[8,11,14]

Nonhormonal copper intrauterine devices (Cu-IUDs) are also safe to use but may be associated with unpredictable vaginal spotting, heavy periods and dysmenorrhoea, which may not be at all desirable.[8,9]

Reversible methods: oral. POP also do not interfere with the gender affirmation hormones.[9] levonorgestrel or norethisterone are the most androgenic progestogens, but as a POP, they only have 3-hour window for late pills and thus may be difficult to comply. The desogestrel POP is a good oral option because of longer administration window of 12 hours. There is a possibility of irregular bleeding with an oral method, which may be unacceptable to a trans male, and it is important to discuss this during counselling.[9,12]

Use of CHC such as pills, patches or the vaginal ring containing oestrogen and progestogen are not recommended if on testosterone treatment, as the oestrogen component of CHC will counteract the masculinising effects of testosterone.[9] This is caused by the fact that CHC can lower androgen levels produced by the ovary and increase sex hormone-binding globulin, which can bind to testosterone thus lowering free testosterone levels.[8]

Permanent methods. Discussion about sterilisation should include stressing the irreversibility of the method and risk of regret especially in those under 30 years.[8,16] Permanent contraception (sterility) can be achieved with tubal occlusion or vasectomy in either partner.[1,9]

Emergency contraception. Trans men and nonbinary (assigned female at birth) people should be offered EC after unprotected vaginal intercourse or if their regular contraception has been compromised or used incorrectly if they do not wish to conceive. Both oral EC methods, (UPA 30 mg and LNG 1.5 mg) and the Cu-IUD, which is the most effective method of EC, can be used without interfering with the gender affirming hormone regimens.[9]

The efficacy of EC is not affected by testosterone.[9] They should be advised to have a urinary pregnancy test 3 weeks after UPSI.[8,17]

Because oral EC does not provide contraceptive cover for subsequent UPSI, trans men and nonbinary will need to use contraception or abstain from sex to avoid further risk of pregnancy.[9]

Contraception for trans people assigned male at birth

Trans women and nonbinary (assigned male at birth) people who have not undergone orchidectomy or vasectomy should ensure that effective contraception is used if they are having vaginal sex with a risk of pregnancy and their partner does not wish to conceive. They can use condoms as a nonpermanent form of contraception with the additional benefit of protection against STIs.[9]

A trans woman or nonbinary person who is receiving oestradiol therapy should be aware that although oestradiol treatment results in impaired spermatogenesis, it does not provide adequate contraceptive protection if they are having vaginal sex. If they are receiving hormonal therapy like GnRH analogues, finasteride or cyproterone acetate, they should be aware that these treatments cannot be relied on for contraceptive protection in terms of reducing or blocking sperm production, and hence there is a risk of pregnancy.[9]

Permanent contraception (sterility) can be achieved with vasectomy.[9]

General gynaecologic problems

Trans men without gender-affirming surgery

Trans men and nonbinary people who have a uterus should be recommended cervical screening which should be undertaken in an appropriate environment and in a sensitive manner. In trans men, there is a 10-fold increased rate of inadequate cytology because of the effect of testosterone on the cervical epithelium. HPV testing could provide reassurance in these cases.[2,9]

Because most trans men are on long-term GnRH analogues and testosterone replacement that may cause amenorrhoea, menstrual-related problems are fairly uncommon. However, if ovarian activity is not adequately suppressed, progestogens, such as norethisterone or medroxyprogesterone, can be used to cause amenorrhoea.[2]

However, any abnormal menstrual bleeding in previously amenorrhoeic individuals on testosterone, should be promptly investigated to rule out endometrial hyperplasia.[2]

Trans men with gender-affirming surgery

Trans men who have had bilateral salpingo-oophorectomy can stop GnRH analogues, as this operation will stop endogenous oestrogen production and improve efficacy of testosterone therapy.[2]

Trans men are eligible for breast screening if they have breast tissue left after bilateral mastectomy.[2]

Pregnancy in trans men

Trans men who have not undergone GAS can become pregnant once they discontinue testosterone treatment, as menstruation will return in most cases. Pregnancy outcomes and complications do not seem to differ much from the general population.

Because of gender dysphoria, feelings of loneliness and isolation can be experienced more during pregnancy. Hence it is important to particularly ensure that they receive individualised care.

Trans women after gender-affirming surgery

Trans women who have undergone GAS may have problems like vaginal discharge, dyspareunia, a 'short' vagina, vaginal hair, voiding difficulties or a lack of lubrication.[2]

Trans women who are on long-term oestrogen therapy are eligible for breast cancer screening.[2]

General sexual health

HIV prevalence rate was 19% in trans women as per a world wide meta-analysis study. The odds ratio was 48.8 of a trans woman being infected with HIV, compared with the general population.[2]

To reduce the risk of HPV-associated cancers, HPV vaccination should be considered for transgender and nonbinary individuals. They should be advised on the importance of using condoms and on vaccination against Hepatitis A and B if engaging in anal sex. Those who engage in high-risk sexual behaviours like chem sex should be advised on the importance of safe sex and the availability of HIV pre-exposure prophylaxis and HIV post-exposure prophylaxis following sexual exposure.[9]

Hormone treatment in transgender people

Hormone preparations used in transgender medicine for gender dysphoria are the same that are used in gonadal endocrinology, although they are not licensed for this use.[18]

The aims of hormone treatment in adult transgender people are to remove as much as possible the earlier effects of the sex steroids of their sex at birth and to induce the desired secondary sex characteristics of the experienced gender. The primary goals of the hormone treatment are usually a degree of feminisation or masculinisation as specified by the patient and this is usually achieved after 2 to 5 years.[18]

Hormone treatment for trans women

Oestrogen. For trans women, recommended oestrogen is the natural form of oestrogen, 17 β-oestradiol, as ethinyl oestradiol, commonly used in oral contraceptives, has been associated with an increase in the risk of venous thromboembolism (VTE) and cardiovascular disease.[18]

Although oestrogen therapy for trans women does not significantly increase risk of VTE, transdermal oestrogen should be used in cases where there are additional risk factors for VTE.[2,18]

The incidence of breast cancer in transwomen using oestrogen therapy has been reported to be the same as the background rate of breast cancer in males.[2]

Prolonged oestrogen therapy leads to a reduction in testicular volume and poor-quality sperm.[2]

Antiandrogen. Monitoring for testosterone and dihydrotestosterone levels is required to ensure adequate suppression is achieved to well below the normal male range. Secretion of the circulating adrenal androgens, androstenedione and dehydroepiandrosterone, will not be suppressed because of the therapy. They have low androgen potency but can be converted to testosterone and dihydrotestosterone. If necessary, their effects may be blocked by the use of finasteride, which inhibits the conversion of testosterone to the more active dihydrotestosterone.[2]

A low dose of the androgen receptor blockers like cyproterone acetate or spironolactone can be started if effects of androgenisation persist. If these agents are used, patients should be counselled regarding monitoring required and potential side effects, such as hepatotoxicity.[5,18]

If trans women have undergone orchidectomy as part of GAS, antiandrogen treatment could be stopped.[18]

Clinical effect. Combined oestrogen and antiandrogen treatment can lead to feminine physical characteristics such as breast development, softer skin, broader hips, and so on. Sometimes additional measures are needed to achieve the desired effects, for example breast augmentation/waxing.[2,18]

Hormone treatment for trans men

Testosterone. In trans men, antioestrogens are not needed. Only testosterone is needed to cause masculine physical characteristics. Testosterone is converted to oestradiol by aromatase activity in fat cells both in men and women. This oestradiol plays an important role in bone physiology in cis men and trans men.[18]

Testosterone therapy usually leads to anovulation and reversible amenorrhea and cessation of monthly periods.[2] The ovarian follicles are not depleted but follicular growth may be affected.[2] For this reason, suitable contraception is still required.

After the gonads have been removed, the goal of the hormone treatment is to avoid hypogonadism and prevent bone loss.[18]

Clinical effect. Testosterone leads to masculine features like increase in lean body mass and muscle strength, body and hair growth, and lowering of the voice.[18]

Development of polycythaemia is a serious risk because testosterone induces the production of erythropoietin. Polycythaemia can lead to cerebrovascular accident, and so it is important to ensure that serum testosterone is at the lower end of the normal range before giving the next dose. However, if polycythaemia develops, venesection can be used in refractory cases.[2,18]

KEY POINTS

- Gender-affirming language, care and support have been shown to improve transgender patient experience in counselling

- Regardless of where a patient identifies on the gender spectrum, they should be provided with up-to-date knowledge of the contraceptive options and management best for them

- Clinician should balance transgender individual's fertility desire in conjunction with contraceptive counselling in discussion; it is important to ascertain use of gender affirming hormones and any previous gender-affirming surgery before discussing contraceptive options for transgender people

- Testosterone in trans men, although causing amenorrhoea, does not provide contraceptive cover; hence there is a need for effective contraception

- Testosterone does not interfere with emergency contraception (EC); EC (copper intrauterine device [IUD]/emergency hormonal contraception) is needed for trans men after unprotected vaginal intercourse if they do not wish to conceive

- Testosterone is teratogenic, and if pregnancy happens, it can cause masculinisation in female foetus

- For trans men on testosterone, combined hormonal contraception (CHC) will affect the masculinising effect of testosterone and hence should not be used; all other methods including progestogen-only pill, DMPA, IUS, IUD and subdermal implant do not interfere with gender-affirming hormones and so can be used safely for contraception

- Rules for quick start after EC for trans men and nonbinary remain same as for cis women except CHC is not used if on testosterone

- Gonadotrophin-releasing hormone agonists, oestrogen and antiandrogens do not provide contraception; therefore there is a need for adequate contraception in partners of trans women

- The UK medical eligibility criteria from the Faculty of Sexual & Reproductive Health care provides important resource with regards to safety of use of a method of contraception with a particular medical condition or personal characteristic when discussing contraceptive options[19]

References

1. Francis A, Jasani S, Bachmann G. Contraceptive challenges and the transgender individual. Womens Midlife Health 2018;4(12).
2. Price S, McManus J, Barrett J. The transgender population: improving awareness for gynaecologists and their role in the provision of care. Obstet Gynaecol 2019;21(1):11–20.
3. Portal.e-lfh.org.uk. Gender Variance. 2016. https://portal.e-lfh.org.uk/Component/Details/438493. Accessed March 30, 2020.
4. The World Professional Association for Transgender Health. Standards of Care for the health of Transsexual, Transgender, and Gender-Nonconforming People. 7th version. WPATH;2012. Available at:https://www.wpath.org/publications/soc [Accessed 2 April 2020].
5. BMJ EBM Spotlight. Gender-affirming hormone in children and adolescents. 2019. https://blogs.bmj.com/bmjebmspotlight/2019/02/25/gender-affirming-hormone-in-children-and-adolescents-evidence-review/. Accessed April 02, 2020.
6. Light A, Wang L, Zeymo A, Gomez-Lobo V. Family planning and contraception use in transgender men. Contraception 2018;98(4):266–269.
7. Jones K, Wood M, Stephens L. Contraception choices for transgender males. J Fam Plann Reprod Health Care 2017;(43):239–240.
8. Krempasky C, Harris M, Abern L, Grimstad F. Contraception across the transmasculine spectrum. Am J Obstet Gynecol 2019;222(2):134–143.
9. FSRH. FSRH CEU statement: contraceptive choices and sexual health for transgender and non-binary people. 2017. https://www.fsrh.org/standards-and-guidance/documents/fsrh-ceu-statement-contraceptive-choices-and-sexual-health-for/ [Accessed 30 March 2020].
10. Trussell J, Aiken ARA. Contraceptive efficacy. In: Hatcher RA, Nelson AL, Trussell J, Cwiak C, Cason P, Policar MS, Edelman A, Aiken ARA, Marrazzo J, Kowal D, eds. Contraceptive technology. 21st ed. New York, NY: Ayer Company Publishers, Inc., 2018.
11. Pfizer Limited emc. Depo-Provera 150mg/ml Injection Sterile Suspension For Injection. 2020. https://www.medicines.org.uk/emc/product/6721/smpc. Accessed April 05, 2020.
12. Lupin Healthcare (UK) Ltd emc. *Desogestrel 75 Microgram Film Coated Tablet.* 2020. https://www.medicines.org.uk/emc/product/7155/smpc. Accessed April 01, 2020.
13. FSRH. FSRH: Intrauterine Contraception. 2015. https://www.fsrh.org/standards-and-guidance/documents/ceuguidanceintrauterinecontraception/. Accessed April 02, 2020.
14. Merck Sharp & Dohme Limited emc. Nexplanon 68 Mg implant for subdermal use. 2020. https://www.medicines.org.uk/emc/product/5720/smpc. Accessed April 05, 2020.
15. Kanj R, Conard L, Trotman G. Menstrual suppression and contraceptive choices in a transgender adolescent and young adult population. J Pediatr Adolesc Gynecol 2016;29(2):201–202.

16. FSRH. FSRH: male and female sterilisation. 2014. https://www.fsrh.org/standards-and-guidance/documents/cec-ceu-guidance-sterilisation-cpd-sep-2014/. Accessed April 02, 2020.

17. FSRH. FSRH guideline: emergency contraception. 2017. https://www.fsrh.org/standards-and-guidance/documents/ceu-clinical-guidance-emergency-contraception-march-2017/. Accessed April 03, 2020.

18. den Heijer M, Bakker A, Gooren L. Long term hormonal treatment for transgender people. BMJ 2017;359(8132):j5027.

19. FSRH. UK medical eligibility criteria for contraceptive use. 2016. https://www.fsrh.org/standards-and-guidance/documents/ukmec-2016/. Accessed March 26, 2020.

Human Immunodeficiency Virus and Contraception

RUPA KUMAR • RUDIGER PITTROF

Case

Precious is 32 years old. She and her husband are from East Africa and came to the United Kingdom 12 years ago. They now run a successful small business and employ five people. Seven years ago, during her first pregnancy Precious was diagnosed with human immunodeficiency virus (HIV) and her husband tested HIV negative. Her HIV has been controlled on treatment with tenofovir disoproxil fumarate/emtricitabine/efavirenz (Atripla®). Her HIV viral load has been undetectable for over 6 years, and her two children are HIV negative. Her husband tests yearly for HIV and has remained HIV negative. Her youngest child, now 1 year old, was conceived following a condom accident. Precious thinks she might want one more child but not in the next year or two, and she requests a more effective method than condoms, particularly as she now knows that U=U (U=U means that people with HIV taking antiretroviral therapy who achieve and maintain an undetectable viral load cannot sexually transmit the virus to others[1]). She is a non-smoker, has no other medical history and no relevant family history. She is not on any other medications. Her blood pressure (BP) is 118/68 mm of Hg, and her body mass index (BMI) is 25 kg/m².

Management

Precious, like anyone, has the right to determine the size of her family. Contraceptive choice can be made independently of her HIV status. However, there are small differences, and it is very important to communicate clearly.

A few antiretroviral medications can reduce the efficacy of certain hormonal contraceptives, which could affect the choice of contraception. Efavirenz can potentially reduce the efficacy of the implant, combined hormonal methods, progestogen-only pill

(POP) and emergency hormonal contraception. Efavirenz does not have any clinically significant effect on efficacy of depo-medroxyprogesterone acetate (DMPA), but the combination may not be ideal for her bone health, as both Tenofovir disoproxil fumarate and DMPA independently lower bone density. Intrauterine contraception ([IUC]: intrauterine device [IUD]/intrauterine system [IUS]) would be the most suitable option for her and should be recommended. However, if the IUD/IUS/DMPA are not acceptable to Precious, she should be advised to use condoms as an additional form of contraception if choosing any of the other hormonal contraceptives. Alternatively, consider referring her back to her HIV clinician to review whether an alternative antiretroviral (ARV) medication could be used instead of efavirenz, to increase her contraceptive choices.

Background

Globally in 2019, an estimated 19.2 million women (aged ≥15 years) were living with HIV, constituting 53% of all adults living with HIV.[2] Women of reproductive age constitute a significant proportion of these individuals. Their need for contraception is poorly met, leading to unplanned pregnancies, vertical transmission, and infant and maternal morbidity and mortality.[3] The World Health Organisation (WHO) recognises the public health importance of providing effective contraception to women living with and at high risk of HIV.[4]

In rich countries, unmet contraceptive needs of women with HIV is less well researched. Women with HIV have regular contact with healthcare providers but may not be given good contraceptive advice. Part of this is caused by misperception that everything to do with HIV, including contraception in women, is difficult and something for specialists.

When helping women with HIV make contraceptive choices, key considerations include drug interactions, efficacy of contraceptives, toxicity and risk of transmission of sexually transmitted infections (STIs) and HIV.[5]

Current evidence suggests that hormonal contraception or IUDs do not increase the risk of HIV acquisition, and that people with an undetectable HIV viral load (indicating that their HIV treatment is fully effective) cannot transmit the virus through sex or from mother to child.

The WHO "Medical eligibility criteria for contraceptive use" (MEC) (2019) states that women at high risk of HIV infection and women with HIV can use any form of reversible hormonal contraception without any restrictions, including progestogen-only injectables, implants and IUDs. However, some ARV medications may reduce the effectiveness of hormonal implants[6] (as well as some other hormonal contraceptives).

The single most important aspect of contraception and HIV is empowerment. We need to empower providers to offer contraception to women with HIV just as they would do to any other woman, and we need to empower women to realise their human right to control their fertility.

Risk of acquisition, transmission and progression of human immunodeficiency virus

The ECHO study, a very large randomised controlled trial comparing HIV incidence in women in Southern and Eastern Africa using progestogen-only injectables, implants and IUDs, found no significant differences in HIV incidence between the different methods.[7]

Some observational studies have suggested a possible increased risk of HIV with progestogen-only injectable use, which was most likely because of unmeasured confounding.[8] The use of DMPA is classed as WHO MEC 1[8], UK MEC 1[9] and US MEC 1[10] (i.e., no restrictions) for women at high risk of HIV.

A WHO Contraceptive Research and Development (CONRAD) technical consultation concluded that vaginal spermicides, such a nonoxynol-9, should not be recommended to women at high risk of HIV infection.[11] There is no evidence of benefit but some evidence of harm by increasing the frequency of genital lesions,[12] and frequent use may increase risk of HIV acquisition.[13] It seems advisable for women with HIV or at high risk of HIV to avoid using spermicides.[14] The use of spermicides and diaphragm are classed as WHO MEC 4[15] and US MEC 4[10] in individuals at high risk of HIV.

Consistent correct condom use is the only proven contraceptive method that reduces risk of HIV transmission,[16] as well as transmission of other STIs. However, condom contraceptive typical use failure rate is 13% in the first year of use.[17] 'Dual protection' should thus be advocated, consisting of barrier contraception to prevent STIs plus a more effective contraceptive to prevent pregnancy.[18]

Women at high risk of acquiring HIV should be offered condoms and HIV preexposure prophylaxis (PrEP), as well as regular (3–12 monthly) HIV testing, STI screening and partner testing.[8] If sex at high risk of transmitting HIV occurred in the last 72 hours, HIV postexposure prophylaxis (PEP) should be discussed too. PEP (typically tenofovir/emtricitabine/raltegravir) and PrEP (typically tenofovir/emtricitabine) have no relevant interactions which will affect the effectiveness of hormonal contraception.

The course of HIV disease is not affected by any method of hormonal contraception[19] or by intrauterine contraceptive devices.[20]

Drug interactions

Top tips

1. **Check out the Liverpool HIV drug interaction data base:**[21]

   https://www.hiv-druginteractions.org/

   It provides a fantastic summary of all interactions between contraceptive drugs and antiretroviral drugs.

2. **Watch out for efavirenz**

   Efavirenz was one of the most common antiretroviral drugs and is still used by many patients taking HIV medicines. It is often part of a fixed-dose combination drug and may not be called efavirenz.

   Efavirenz induces the hepatic enzyme CYP3A4. This is an enzyme that also metabolizes hormonal contraceptives. When they are co-administered, efavirenz results in a more rapid clearance of progestogens and has a variable effect on ethinyl oestradiol levels with different formulations. It may also decrease the bioavailability of ulipristal acetate (UPA).[21] Efavirenz does not make hormonal contraceptives dangerous but makes some of them less effective.

3. **Watch out for protease inhibitors**

   Protease inhibitors atazanavir, darunavir, lopinavir, cobicistat and ritonavir induce or inhibit enzymes and affect drug levels for contraceptive hormones. This may make contraception less effective. It is important to avoid prescribing drospirenone-containing contraceptives to patients taking atazanavir + cobicistat, as this can cause hyperkalaemia. If your patient is on a protease inhibitor, use the Liverpool HIV drug interaction data base[21] to look it up. Protease inhibitors are often included in fixed dose combination medications and will have a different trade name.

4. **Watch out for antibiotics for tuberculosis**

   Patients may be taking potent enzyme (CYP3A) inducers, such as rifampicin (for *Mycobacterium tuberculosis*) and rifabutin (for *Mycobacterium avium intracellulare*), to treat HIV-associated complications or comorbidities. All these enzyme-inducing agents can cause hormonal contraception failure up to 4 weeks following completion of treatment.[22]

Contraceptive choices in human immunodeficiency virus

What is different for women taking antiretroviral medication who need emergency contraception?

Just a little! Women who request emergency contraception (EC) should be offered the choice of emergency IUD insertion or oral emergency contraception. However, some ARV medications are enzyme inducers and may theoretically reduce the effectiveness of oral emergency contraception: notably efavirenz. It results in a more rapid clearance of levonorgestrel[23] and possibly Ulipristal.[21] Management advice is to use levonorgestrel 3 mg single dose (double the licensed dose) if oral emergency contraception requested, irrespective of the patient's weight or BMI.[24] Use of double dose of UPA-EC is not recommended.[24] However, the IUD would be the most effective emergency contraceptive.

What is different for women taking antiretroviral medication requesting short-acting reversible contraception?

Just a little! Short-acting reversible contraception (SARC) includes the combined oral contraceptive, combined hormonal patch and vaginal ring and progestogen-only pill (POP). Women who request SARC should be recommended a long-acting reversible contraception (LARC) method because of the superior effectiveness of LARC. In a randomised controlled trial, Hubacher et al. (2017)[25] showed that for women requesting short-acting methods but in equipoise about using a LARC method, 1-year pregnancy rates in those randomised to SARC and LARC were 7.7% and 0.7%, respectively. These women were not HIV positive, but there is no reason to expect a different outcome for women who are on HIV treatment. Interactions between most HIV medications and hormonal contraceptives are not clinically significant. There are two main exceptions: efavirenz makes SARCs less effective, and the combination of atazanavir/cobicistat (Evotaz®) with drospirenone can cause dangerous hyperkalaemia.

- **If your patient cannot remember what she is taking for her HIV:** use any bridging method, for example, desogestrel 75 mcg POP (assuming no other contraindications) backed up by condoms until she had a chance to inform you of her HIV drugs or discuss her contraception with her HIV care provider. Studies suggest that contraceptives will not make her HIV treatment less effective.[26] Her HIV treatment might affect her SARC, but some contraception is always better than no contraception at all.

- **If your patient is on efavirenz:** SARCs are not a good option. Decreases in contraceptive hormone levels in women taking combined oral contraceptives (COCs) were seen in pharmaco-kinetic studies suggesting potential for contraceptive failure.[27,28] Taken together with being a user-dependent method relying on adherence, oral contraception may not be the most effective option.[26] There is no restriction on the use of SARCs for non-contraceptive purposes.

- **If your patient is on a protease inhibitor (PI):** protease in-hibitors reduce ethinylestradiol (EE) levels with the exception of atazanavir/cobicistat and atazanavir without ritonavir. Some studies have reported increased progestin levels when certain PIs are used with hormonal contraceptives,[29,30] but these changes are unlikely to impact safety.[26] A systematic review by Nanda et al (2017) found that despite the observed decreased EE plasma levels, concurrent use of protease inhibitors with COCs does not alter contraceptive effectiveness, as the progestin component is primarily responsible for contraceptive effective-ness. It is thought that in combined hormonal contraception the progestogen inhibits ovulation by blocking the midcycle luteinising hormone surge, while the oestrogen component prevents irregular bleeding.[31]

- **If your patient is using HIV drugs that are not protease inhibitors or efavirenz:** no change in management unless she is on an integrase inhibitor called *elvitegravir/cobicistat* which reduces EE levels (advice: use COC preparations containing at least 30 mcg EE).

None of the studies were of adequate quality to provide the guidance that providers and HIV-infected women need when con-sidering contraceptive options. High-quality, well-powered studies are required to address the efficacy of hormonal contraception when coadministered with antiretroviral therapy (ART).

Other considerations

Some ARVs—for example, efavirenz and PIs—are associated with metabolic side effects. Patients with HIV have higher rates of smok-ing and are at increased risk of coronary artery disease compared with the general population.[32] Evidence has suggested combined hormonal contraception may increase risk of myocardial infarction and thrombotic stroke.[33] When considering hormonal contraception, clinicians should consider the potential complications that may results from these additive risks.[34]

The COC is metabolized by the liver. It is contraindicated in severe (decompensated) cirrhosis (UK medical eligibility criteria [MEC] 4). Initiation of combined oral contraception in acute or flare-up of viral hepatitis is classed as UKMEC 3.[9] This is of relevance, as patients with HIV may have concurrent hepatitis (alcohol related/viral) or ARV related liver damage. Patients with HIV may be intravenous drug users with chronic active hepatitis C infection. (Note: these individuals may have a chaotic lifestyle; thus user-dependent contraceptives may not be a reliable option.[14]) Albeit to a lesser extent than COCs, progestogen-only contraceptives may adversely affect patients with impaired liver function (because these are also metabolised by the liver).[9]

The concept of the 'pill burden' of highly active antiretroviral therapy is widely acknowledged, leading to poor adherence.[35,36] This is worth discussing with patients when considering oral contraceptives; a non-daily, non-oral contraceptive may be preferable.[37]

What is different for women taking antiretroviral medication requesting long-acting hormonal contraception?

Almost nothing! Women who request a LARC method should get the method of their choice. However, there are a few important things to consider:

1. **Implant and efavirenz:**

   Efavirenz (and possibly Nevirapine) reduces the effectiveness of implants. In a recently published retrospective cohort study from Kenya, pregnancy incidence in women taking efavirenz-based ART was 4.78 per 100-person years for levonorgestrel implants, and 10 per 100-person years for etonogestrel implants. Nevirapine use was associated with a similar rate of pregnancy. There were no pregnancies recorded in women on PI-based regimens.[38] Numerous case reports have shown contraceptive failure in women taking efavirenz. It is thus imperative to counsel women taking efavirenz of the importance of dual contraception.[37]

2. **DMPA injections and efavirenz:**

   The pharmacokinetics and efficacy of DMPA did not appear to be altered in the presence of efavirenz.[21,39,40] However, a study from Malawi in 2019 showed significantly lower concentrations of MPA (medroxyprogesterone acetate) in HIV-positive African women on efavirenz- or nevirapine-based ART regimens compared with HIV-negative women.[41]

Use of MPA by women with HIV-associated tuberculosis (TB) receiving efavirenz and rifampicin resulted in more rapid clearance of MPA, leading to subtherapeutic concentrations of MPA in some women at 10 and 12 weeks postinjection. However, there was no increase in progesterone concentrations, suggesting ovulation unlikely to have occurred.[42] The authors suggested a more frequent dosing (8–10 weekly) to avert potential contraceptive failure in this group of women.

There is lack of evidence on whether the lower-dose subcutaneous MPA might be susceptible to drug interactions.[21]

3. **Bone and HIV:**

People living with HIV/AIDS are at increased risk of osteoporosis. Some antiretroviral drugs, particularly tenofovir and PIs, have been implicated in this.[43] This risk should be considered before prescribing MPA injections, which are also associated with increased risk of osteoporosis. There are good alternatives to these ARVs.

4. **IUS/IUD and infection risk:**

IUC is safe and effective in HIV-infected women.[44] There appears to be no increased risk of infectious complications with use of IUC, nor has it been found to adversely affect HIV progression or transmission to sexual partners.[20]

Women who have a low CD4 ($<200/mm^3$) count or severe/advanced HIV clinical disease may be at increased risk of pelvic inflammatory disease following IUD or IUS insertion, and IUD/IUS insertion is classified as UKMEC 3,[9] WHO MEC 3[15] and US MEC 2.[10] A "3" classification implies that the theoretical or proven risks usually outweigh the advantages of using the method. The provision of a method requires expert clinical judgement and/or referral to a specialist contraceptive provider, because use of the method is not usually recommended unless other more appropriate methods are not available or not acceptable. The evidence base for this recommendation is not clear (Tepper et al 2016).[20] Immunosuppressed patients with HIV who request an IUD/IUS insertion should have tests for STIs at the time of insertion and should be informed of the symptoms of pelvic inflammatory disease (PID) and what to do if they are suspected.

What to do if her contraceptive choice does not work well with her antiretroviral regime?

There are many excellent treatment options for HIV. A patient does not have to be on efavirenz. Efavirenz is no longer a preferred WHO (2019) or British HIV Association (2015)[45] choice when starting HIV treatment. Effective and comfortable contraception is as important as good HIV control. If a specific method of contraception would enhance the quality of life of a patient much more than any other but would interact with the HIV medication, it is entirely appropriate to contact the HIV care provider and suggest to review her HIV medication.

What is different for women taking antiretroviral medication requesting permanent contraception?

Absolutely nothing. Any woman has the right to choose permanent contraception; we need to ensure that she is not pressurised into making this decision. Sterilisation procedure and success are not affected by her HIV status.

Pregnancy planning and human immunodeficiency virus

Contraception is only one part of family planning. People with HIV have a chronic condition, and just like anyone with a chronic health problem, they may wish to achieve their ideal family size before their health or age makes it harder to do so. It is our task as sexual healthcare providers to enable them to do so. Pregnancy planning should include a visit to the HIV clinic to optimise HIV-related health before pregnancy. Efavirenz and dolutegravir are considered safe in pregnancy, but some doubt remains about their potential to cause neurodevelopmental deficits and neural tube defects,[47] respectively.

Postpartum contraception

In affluent countries, postpartum women with HIV should not breastfeed to reduce risk of vertical transmission to the infant. Without the lactational amenorrhea contraceptive method, women should be offered contraception in the postpartum period to reduce risk of unplanned pregnancy.

Conclusion

A woman taking antiretrovirals for HIV treatment or prevention has the same sexual and reproductive health rights as any other woman. She should therefore have access to the full range of contraceptive options and be enabled to make informed decisions about her options.[26] Contraceptive efficacy of some hormonal contraceptives is likely to be reduced for women taking efavirenz or nevirapine, and possibly for those taking protease inhibitors. Contraceptive efficacy may be reduced by certain antibiotics for HIV-associated diseases, such as TB. Further large-scale prospective studies using clinical outcomes, such as ovulation and pregnancy rates during long-term administration, rather than pharmacokinetic data, are required to better establish interactions between contraceptives and ART agents in combination. This knowledge will better inform guidelines to help support the sexual and reproductive rights of women living with and at risk of HIV.[26]

Contraceptive efficacy is only one of many factors that an individual may consider when choosing a contraceptive method, and an adequately informed woman with HIV should be free to choose any hormonal or non-hormonal permanent or reversible method of contraception even if there is concern for decreased efficacy when used with efavirenz.[26] In real-life setting, user-independent contraceptive implants are more effective than user-dependent methods, including DMPA, despite a reduced effectiveness when used with efavirenz.[48] We have a right and the duty to ask HIV care providers to review the HIV treatment regime if this would improve the quality of life of our patient (e.g., by enabling her to use her preferred method of contraception).

KEY POINTS

- A woman taking antiretrovirals for HIV treatment or prevention has the same sexual and reproductive health rights as any other woman; she should therefore have access to the full range of contraceptive options and be enabled to make informed decisions about her options

- Current evidence states that contraceptive methods do not increase risk of acquisition, transmission or progression of HIV

- Spermicides should not be used in patients at high risk of HIV

- Condoms are the only contraceptive method that prevents transmission of HIV and sexually transmitted infections (STIs) and should always be recommended to patients at high STI/HIV risk

- Drug interactions occur between contraceptives and some antiretroviral (ARV) medications; check the Liverpool HIV drug interaction database[21] before prescribing contraceptives to patients on antiretroviral drugs

- Efavirenz reduces efficacy of oral emergency contraception, combined hormonal contraceptives, progestogen-only pill and implants; dual contraception (condoms) should be recommended to these patients; intrauterine device (IUD)/intrauterine system (IUS)/depo-medroxyprogesterone acetate are suitable options. You can consider referral to a HIV specialist to suggest an alternative ARV regimen

- Beware of interactions between antibiotics for tuberculosis and some hormonal contraceptives; note that the effect may persist up to 4 weeks after completion of antibiotic treatment

- Consider metabolic, cardiovascular and osteoporosis risk of ARVs when prescribing contraceptives

- Immunosuppressed patients with HIV who have an IUD/IUS inserted should have tests for STIs at the time of insertion and should be informed of the symptoms of pelvic inflammatory disease and what to do if they are suspected

- All women, including those with HIV, should be offered contraception in the postpartum period to reduce risk of unplanned pregnancy

- Further research using outcomes, such as ovulation and pregnancy rates, rather than pharmacokinetic data, are required to better establish interactions between contraceptives and antiretroviral therapy

References

1. Eisinger RW, Dieffenbach CW, Fauci AS. HIV viral load and transmissibility of HIV infection: undetectable equals untransmittable. JAMA 2019;321(5):451–452.
2. UNAIDS AIDS info. Global Factsheets 2019. 2019. http://aidsinfo.unaids.org/.

3. Johnston B, Ligiero D, DeSilva S, Medley A, Nightingale V, Sripipatana T, et al. Meeting the family planning needs of women living with HIV in US government global health programs. AIDS 2013;27 Suppl 1(1):S121–S125.
4. The Inter-agency Task Team for Prevention and Treatment of HIV Infection in Pregnant Women, Mothers, and their Children. Preventing HIV and unintended pregnancies: strategic framework 2011–2015. World Health Organization; 2012. https://www.who.int/reproductivehealth/publications/linkages/hiv_pregnancies_2012/en/.
5. Sharma M, Walmsley SL. Contraceptive options for HIV-positive women: making evidence-based, patient-centred decisions. HIV Med 2015;16(6):329–336.
6. World Health Organization. Women and adolescent girls living with HIV need better advice and access to contraceptives. World Health Organization; 2019. https://www.who.int/hiv/mediacentre/news/contraceptive-for-women-girl-living-with-hiv/en/.
7. Evidence for Contraceptive Options and HIV Outcomes (ECHO) Trial Consortium, Ahmed K, Baeten JM, Beksinska M, Bekker LG, Bukusi EA, et al. HIV incidence among women using intramuscular depot medroxyprogesterone acetate, a copper intrauterine device, or a levonorgestrel implant for contraception: a randomised, multicentre, open-label trial. Lancet 2019;394(10195):303–313.
8. World Health Organization. Contraceptive eligibility for women at high risk of HIV: Guidance statement - Recommendations on contraceptive methods used by women at high risk of HIV. 2019. https://apps.who.int/iris/bitstream/handle/10665/326653/9789241550574-eng.pdf?ua=1.
9. Faculty of Sexual & Reproductive Healthcare. UK Medical Eligibility Criteria for Contraceptive Use: UKMEC 2016 (amended September 2019). 2016. https://www.fsrh.org/standards-and-guidance/documents/ukmec-2016/.
10. Centers for Disease Control and Prevention (CDC), US Medical Eligiblity Criteria (US MEC) for Contraceptive Use. Summary of classifications for hormonal contraceptive methods and intrauterine devices. 2016. https://www.cdc.gov/reproductivehealth/contraception/mmwr/mec/appendixk.html#mec_hiv.
11. World Health Organization, Department of Reproductive Health and Research. WHO/CONRAD Technical Consultation on Nonoxynol-9. Geneva: WHO; October 2001: Summary Report, 2001. https://www.who.int/reproductivehealth/publications/rtis/RHR_03_8/en/.
12. Wilkinson D, Ramjee G, Tholandi M, Rutherford G. Nonoxynol-9 for preventing vaginal acquisition of HIV infection by women from men. Cochrane Database Syst Rev 2002;(4):CD003936.
13. Van Damme L, Ramjee G, Alary M, Vuylsteke B, Chandeying V, Rees H, et al., COL-1492 Study Group. Effectiveness of COL-1492, a nonoxynol-9 vaginal gel, on HIV-1 transmission in female sex workers: a randomised controlled trial. Lancet 2002;360(9338):971–977.
14. Mitchell HS, Stephens E. Contraception choice for HIV positive women. Sex Transm Infect 2004;80(3):167–173.
15. World Health Organization. Medical eligibility criteria for contraceptive use – Fifth Edition. 2015. https://apps.who.int/iris/bitstream/handle/10665/181468/9789241549158_eng.pdf?sequence=9.
16. Davis KR, Weller SC. The effectiveness of condoms in reducing heterosexual transmission of HIV. Fam Plann Perspect 1999;31(6):272–279.
17. Trussell J, Aiken ARA. Contraceptive efficacy. In: Hatcher RA, Nelson AL, Trussell J, Cwiak C, Cason P, Policar MS, Edelman A, Aiken ARA, Marrazzo J, Kowal D, eds. Contraceptive technology. 21st ed. New York, NY: Ayer Company Publishers, Inc., 2018.
18. International Planned Parenthood Federation (IPPF). International Medical Advisory Panel (IMAP) Statement on Expanding Access and Contraceptive Choice through Integrated Sexual and Reproductive Health Services. 2019. https://www.ippf.org/sites/default/files/2019-12/IMAP%20statement%20on%20expanding%20access%20and%20contraceptive%20choice%20through%20integrated%20sexual%20and%20reproductive%20health%20services.pdf.

19. Phillips SJ, Curtis KM, Polis CB. Effect of hormonal contraceptive methods on HIV disease progression: a systematic review. AIDS 2013;27(5):787–794.
20. Tepper NK, Curtis KM, Nanda K, Jamieson DJ. Safety of intrauterine devices among women with HIV: a systematic review. Contraception 2016;94(6):713–724.
21. University of Liverpool. HIV Drug Interactions. 2019. https://liverpool-hiv-hep.s3.amazonaws.com/prescribing_resources/pdfs/000/000/025/original/TS_Contraceptive_2019_Dec.pdf?1576668395; www.hiv-druginteractions.org/Interactions.aspx.
22. Dickinson BD, Altman RD, Nielsen NH, Sterling ML, Council on Scientific Affairs, American Medical Association. Drug interactions between oral contraceptives and antibiotics. Obstet Gynecol 2001;98(5 Pt 1):853–860.
23. Carten ML, Kiser JJ, Kwara A, Mawhinney S, Cu-Uvin S. Pharmacokinetic interactions between the hormonal emergency contraception, levonorgestrel (Plan B), and Efavirenz. Infect Dis Obstet Gynecol 2012;2012:137–192.
24. Faculty of Sexual and Reproductive Healthcare. Emergency Contraception March 2017 (Amended December 2020). https://www.fsrh.org/standards-and-guidance/documents/ceu-clinical-guidance-emergency-contraception-march-2017/.
25. Hubacher D, Spector H, Monteith C, Chen PL, Hart C. Long-acting reversible contraceptive acceptability and unintended pregnancy among women presenting for short-acting methods: a randomized patient preference trial. Am J Obstet Gynecol 2017;216(2):101–109.
26. Nanda K, Stuart GS, Robinson J, Gray AL, Tepper NK, Gaffield ME. Drug interactions between hormonal contraceptives and antiretrovirals. AIDS 2017;31(7):917–952.
27. Landolt NK, Phanuphak N, Ubolyam S, Pinyakorn S, Kriengsinyot R, Ahluwalia J, et al. Efavirenz, in contrast to nevirapine, is associated with unfavorable progesterone and antiretroviral levels when coadministered with combined oral contraceptives. J Acquir Immune Defic Syndr 2013;62(5):534–539.
28. Sevinsky H, Eley T, Persson A, Garner D, Yones C, Nettles R, et al. The effect of efavirenz on the pharmacokinetics of an oral contraceptive containing ethinyl estradiol and norgestimate in healthy HIV-negative women. Antivir Ther 2011;16(2):149–156.
29. DuBois BN, Atrio J, Stanczyk FZ, Cherala G. Increased exposure of norethindrone in HIV+ women treated with ritonavir-boosted atazanavir therapy. Contraception 2015;91(1):71–75.
30. Zhang J, Chung E, Yones C, Persson A, Mahnke L, Eley T, et al. The effect of atazanavir/ritonavir on the pharmacokinetics of an oral contraceptive containing ethinyl estradiol and norgestimate in healthy women. Antivir Ther 2011;16(2):157–164.
31. Rivera R, Yacobson I, Grimes D. The mechanism of action of hormonal contraceptives and intrauterine contraceptive devices. Am J Obstet Gynecol 1999;181(5 Pt 1):1263–1269.
32. Lifson AR, Neuhaus J, Arribas JR, van den Berg-Wolf M, Labriola AM, Read TR, INSIGHT SMART Study Group. Smoking-related health risks among persons with HIV in the Strategies for Management of Antiretroviral Therapy clinical trial. Am J Public Health 2010;100(10):1896–1903.
33. Lidegaard Ø, Løkkegaard E, Jensen A, Skovlund CW, Keiding N. Thrombotic stroke and myocardial infarction with hormonal contraception. N Engl J Med 2012;366(24):2257–2266.
34. Womack J, Richman S, Tien PC, Grey M, Williams A. Hormonal contraception and HIV-positive women: metabolic concerns and management strategies. J Midwifery Womens Health 2008;53(4):362–375.
35. Juday T, Gupta S, Grimm K, Wagner S, Kim E. Factors associated with complete adherence to HIV combination antiretroviral therapy. HIV Clin Trials 2011;12(2):71–78.
36. Atkinson MJ, Petrozzino JJ. An evidence-based review of treatment-related determinants of patients' nonadherence to HIV medications. AIDS Patient Care STDS 2009;23(11):903–914.
37. Robinson JA, Jamshidi R, Burke AE. Contraception for the HIV-positive woman: a review of interactions between hormonal contraception and antiretroviral therapy. Infect Dis Obstet Gynecol 2012;2012:890160.

38. Pfitzer A, Wille J, Wambua J, Stender SC, Strachan M, Ayuyo CM, et al. Contraceptive implant failures among women using antiretroviral therapy in western Kenya: a retrospective cohort study. Gates Open Res 2019;3:1482.

39. Watts DH, Park JG, Cohn SE, Yu S, Hitti J, Stek A, et al. Safety and tolerability of depot medroxyprogesterone acetate among HIV-infected women on antiretroviral therapy: ACTG A5093. Contraception 2008;77(2):84–90.

40. Cohn SE, Park JG, Watts DH, Stek A, Hitti J, Clax PA, et al., ACTG A5093 Protocol Team. Depo-medroxyprogesterone in women on antiretroviral therapy: effective contraception and lack of clinically significant interactions. Clin Pharmacol Ther 2007;81(2):222–227.

41. Zia Y, Tang JH, Chinula L, Tegha G, Stanczyk FZ, Kourtis AP. Medroxyprogesterone acetate concentrations among HIV-infected depot-medroxyprogesterone acetate users receiving antiretroviral therapy in Lilongwe, Malawi. Contraception 2019;100(5):402–405.

42. Mngqibisa R, Kendall MA, Dooley K, Wu XS, Firnhaber C, Mcilleron H, et al., A5338 Study Team. Pharmacokinetics and pharmacodynamics of depot medroxyprogesterone acetate in African women receiving treatment for human immunodeficiency virus and tuberculosis: potential concern for standard dosing frequency. Clin Infect Dis 2020;71(3):517–524.

43. McComsey GA, Tebas P, Shane E, Yin MT, Overton ET, Huang JS, et al. Bone disease in HIV infection: a practical review and recommendations for HIV care providers. Clin Infect Dis 2010;51(8):937–946.

44. Stringer EM, Kaseba C, Levy J, Sinkala M, Goldenberg RL, Chi BH, et al. A randomized trial of the intrauterine contraceptive device vs hormonal contraception in women who are infected with the human immunodeficiency virus. Am J Obstet Gynecol 2007;197(2):144.e1–144.e8.

45. British HIV Association. British HIV Association guidelines for the treatment of HIV-1-positive adults with antiretroviral therapy 2015 (2016 interim update). 2015. https://www.bhiva.org/file/RVYKzFwyxpgil/treatment-guidelines-2016-interim-update.pdf.

46. Cassidy AR, Williams PL, Leidner J, Mayondi G, Ajibola G, Makhema J, et al. In utero efavirenz exposure and neurodevelopmental outcomes in HIV-exposed uninfected children in botswana. Pediatr Infect Dis J. 2019;38(8):828–834.

47. Zash R, Holmes L, Diseko M, Jacobson DL, Brummel S, Mayondi G, et al. Neural-tube defects and antiretroviral treatment regimens in botswana. N Engl J Med 2019;381(9):827–840.

48. Patel RC, Onono M, Gandhi M, Blat C, Hagey J, Shade SB, et al. Pregnancy rates in HIV-positive women using contraceptives and efavirenz-based or nevirapine-based antiretroviral therapy in Kenya: a retrospective cohort study. Lancet HIV 2015;2(11):e474–e482.

Contraception and Mental Health

RUPA KUMAR • RUDIGER PITTROF

Case

Maddie is 25 years old and has recently had a 3-week admission to a mental health (MH) ward following an episode of mania with psychosis. She had unprotected sex with a number of men during this episode. Her pregnancy test was negative both at the start and end of her admission to the ward. Maddie was diagnosed with bipolar affective disorder during admission and was started on olanzapine tablets.

She is presenting to her general practitioner (GP) 2 months after discharge from hospital to request contraception, as her friend suggested she use a more reliable method than condoms alone. She does not have a regular sexual partner. Her last sexual intercourse was with a casual male partner a month ago without a condom. She could not recall the date of her last menstrual period and was expecting her period anytime soon. She had regular monthly periods previously. Maddie has a 3-year-old child from an unplanned pregnancy, and does not wish to have another child for the next few years. She has no other medical problems, is a non-smoker, drinks socially and does not take any other medications or recreational drugs. She has no relevant family history. Her body mass index (BMI) is 29 kg/m^2, and her blood pressure is 124/68 mm Hg.

Management

Bipolar affective disorder (BPAD) is characterised by periods of mania or hypomania, as well as periods of depression.[1] Mainstay of pharmacologic treatment consists of antipsychotics and or mood stabilizers.

In the case of Maddie, firstly, a pregnancy should be excluded. Maddie has no contraindications to any contraceptive, including the combined hormonal contraception. Currently, there is inconsistent evidence to support a link between most hormonal contraceptives and negative impact on mood.[2] Certain mood stabilizers used to treat BPAD can interact with contraceptive methods, and some—notably, sodium valproate, carbamazepine and lithium—are associated with teratogenicity. Patients on teratogenic medications must be on highly effective contraception. Olanzapine is not teratogenic and does not interfere with contraceptive levels in the blood.

Olanzapine is a second-generation antipsychotic associated with metabolic syndrome and increased risk of obesity. Thus combined hormonal contraception may not be the best long-term contraceptive. Depot medroxyprogesterone acetate (DMPA) injections are associated with weight gain. Some antipsychotics are associated with hyperprolactinaemia (less common with olanzapine compared to other antipsychotics),[3–5] increasing risk of osteoporosis. This is worth bearing in mind if considering DMPA contraceptive injections. Oligo/amenorrhea can result from hyperprolactinaemia, which patients may mistakenly perceive to be associated with infertility. Patients should be informed that they are still capable of becoming pregnant.[6]

Mania in BPAD is associated with impulsivity and risky sexual behaviour. Risk of unplanned pregnancy has been shown to be greater in patients with BPAD compared with healthy controls.[7] Unplanned pregnancy increases risk of bipolar disease relapse during pregnancy. Because poor contraceptive adherence is a common problem, a long-acting reversible method of contraception (LARC) should be discussed with Maddie, as LARC methods have been shown to be more effective than short acting reversible contraceptive (SARC) methods in preventing unplanned pregnancies.[8]

Maddie should also be advised to use condoms additionally to prevent sexually transmitted infections (STI) and be offered a full STI screen.

In the future, if Maddie wishes to become pregnant, she should receive preconception counselling about the risks to her health and to her child. BPAD is associated with obesity, metabolic syndrome, diabetes,[9] as well as alcohol and substance misuse, with risks to the mother and foetus. Maddie should be encouraged to achieve a normal BMI before conception. Additionally, she should be provided with folic acid supplementation before pregnancy to reduce the risk of neural tube defects.

Women are particularly vulnerable to relapse during the postpartum period. To reduce risk of relapse, women with BPAD should aim for a period of at least 6 to 24 months of stabilization of their mental illness (euthymia) before planning a pregnancy.[10] Maintenance pharmacotherapy during pregnancy may reduce risk of recurrent mood episodes.[11]

Background

One in five women in England have a common mental disorder, and the rates have been steadily increasing.[12] MH problems are often undiagnosed and untreated in women of reproductive age, and are disproportionately linked with socio-economic deprivation.

Individuals with MH problems are faced with increased risk of adverse sexual and reproductive health outcomes, such as unplanned pregnancies, increased risk of STIs and human immunodeficiency virus, adverse perinatal and postpartum outcomes, teratogenicity associated with psychotropic medications, drugs and alcohol misuse, sexual dysfunction and non-consensual sex. There is also lower prevalence of contraceptive use and adherence.[13] Associated drugs and alcohol misuse can also expose them to risky sexual behaviour. Maternal mental illness and substance misuse are significant risk factors for children being taken into care.[14]

Neglecting sexual and reproductive health (SRH) needs in patients with MH problems has enormous impact on the individual and society. Due to the aforementioned vulnerabilities, people with MH problems find it harder to use SRH services. SRH services are partly to blame for this: processes, such as internet booking, self-assessment and long waiting times can unwittingly filter out patients with MH problems before we see them. SRH needs are also often not addressed in MH settings[15,16]: a study showed that only 25% of professionals raised the topic with patients.[17]

National Institute for Health and Care Excellence guidance (CG192) 2014 (updated 2018) advises that contraception and pregnancy planning, must be discussed with all women of childbearing potential who have a new, existing or past MH problem.[18]

Good SRH care is not all about contraception. It is also about helping individuals to optimise their chances of a healthy pregnancy by providing preconception care.

Considerations for contraceptive choices

Table 26.1 (Kumar and Pathak[19]) show specific SRH issues to consider in different mental illnesses.[19]

User-dependent versus user-independent contraceptives

User-dependent methods of contraception rely on the individual or their partner to remember to use them regularly or during sex.

Table 26.1

SRH Issues In Mental Illness: Considerations	
Mental illness	**Issues to consider**
Bipolar affective disorder	• Impulsivity and risky sexual behaviour associated with mania • Mood stabilisers resulting in drug interactions and teratogenicity
Psychotic disorders	• Delusions associated with indwelling contraception • Antipsychotic-induced hyperprolactinaemia, amenorrhoea or oligomenorrhoea associated with perception of infertility • Metabolic syndrome associated with second generation antipsychotics • Higher rates of cardiovascular disease, obesity and smoking resulting in contraindications to combined hormonal contraception • Mood stabilisers as adjuncts resulting in drug interactions and teratogenicity
Anxiety and depression	• Heightened negative perceptions of contraception and its impact on mood • Impact of fluctuating or low motivation on user-dependent contraceptive methods (condoms, pills, patches, vaginal rings) • St John's wort associated with reduced efficacy of certain hormonal contraceptives
Eating disorders	• Weight gain concerns • Amenorrhoea and a perception of infertility • Return to fertility precedes return of first period, requiring effective contraception to prevent unwanted pregnancy
Substance misuse disorders	• High risk of unplanned pregnancy, risk of foetal exposure to alcohol, drugs, tobacco

(Reproduced with permission from Kumar U, Pathak N. Maudsley Guidelines: Contraception and Mental Health. In: Taylor D, Gaughran F, Pillinger T, editors. The Maudsley: Practice Guidelines for Physical Health Conditions in Psychiatry. London: Wiley Blackwell; 2020. p. 307–316.)

In individuals with serious mental illness, chaotic lifestyles, impulsiveness and poor judgement result in a greater failure rate of these methods.[20] Such methods include barrier contraception, natural family planning, oral contraceptives (combined and progestogen only), vaginal ring, and patch. In addition to other, more reliable contraceptive methods, barrier contraception should be recommended to all individuals to reduce the transmission of STIs.

Nonuser-dependent methods include LARCs and sterilisation. Because the patient does not need to remember to take/use them, LARCs are the most effective forms of contraception and they should routinely be offered to individuals. LARCs include the implant, injection, intrauterine systems (IUS) and copper intrauterine device (Cu-IUD).

Many patients with serious mental illness (SMI) are administered depot psychotropic medications, presenting a potential window of opportunity for contraceptive injections to be administered, if the patient wishes.[20] Patients, however, need to remember to repeat injections at regular intervals.

IUS/IUD devices also offer the advantage of being local contraceptives, thus minimising systemic side effects and drug interactions with psychotropic medications. The Cu-IUD can be used as emergency contraception. A potential drawback of LARCs is that there are reports of indwelling devices having become the focus of delusions in individuals with psychotic illness.[21]

Drug interactions between psychotropic medications and contraceptives

Enzyme-inducing psychotropic medications

Drug interactions with contraceptive hormones frequently occur with antiepileptic or mood-stabilising drugs (e.g., carbamazepine, topiramate), as well as St. John's wort (hypericum perforatum) (an over-the-counter antidepressant therapy). These drugs reduce the bioavailability and efficacy of combined hormonal contraception, progestogen-only pill, contraceptive implant and oral emergency contraception, both during use and for up to 28 days after stopping medication.[20] Patients on these psychotropic medications should be offered the IUD/IUS or DMPA injection instead.

Hormonal contraceptives affecting psychotropic medication levels

1. **Lamotrigine**

   Lamotrigine is an antiepileptic and mood-stabilising drug. It is not an enzyme-inducing drug and does not affect contraceptive effectiveness, but some hormonal contraceptives can affect lamotrigine levels. Combined oral contraception reduced lamotrigine trough levels up to 70%, with potential reduced symptom control. Conversely lamotrigine levels increase twofold during the pill-free interval with potential for toxicity.[22] To keep lamotrigine levels predictable women using combined hormonal contraception should use regimes without a hormone-free interval. Lamotrigine dosing should be reviewed after initiation and discontinuation of combined hormonal contraception. Insufficient data exists on the effect of Progestogen-only methods on Lamotrigine metabolism; Limited evidence suggests Desogestrel POP might increase Lamotrigine levels.[23]

2. **Antipsychotics**

Combined oral contraceptives inhibit the metabolism of clozapine, leading to clozapine levels increasing to almost three times more than the normal plasma concentration. This can lead to hypotension, tremor, sedation and nausea.[24] Combined oral contraceptives affect the antipsychotic chlorpromazine in the same way.[25,26] Stopping combined oral contraception leads to a decrease in clozapine and chlorpromazine levels, requiring antipsychotic dose adjustment to ensure therapeutic levels.

Please see the FSRH guidance on drug interactions for more details.[27]

For up-to-date information on drug interactions, refer to sources such as:

British National Formulary (BNF) (www.bnf.org)[28]

Stockley's Drug Interactions (www.medicinescomplete.com/mc/index.htm)[29]

Electronic Medicine Compendium (www.medicines.org.uk/emc)[30]

Side effects of psychotropic medications

Teratogenicity

The risk of congenital malformations associated with use of antipsychotics and antidepressants during pregnancy is generally low.[31–34] Mood stabilisers, such as sodium valproate, carbamazepine and topiramate, are teratogenic and lithium may increase the risk of congenital malformation in the exposed foetus.[31]

Sodium valproate is highly teratogenic and is associated with major congenital abnormalities (10.3%), poorer neurodevelopmental outcomes, autism low IQ (30%–40%).[35] Valproate must no longer be used in any woman or girl able to have children, unless she has a pregnancy prevention programme in place.[36] Carbamazepine is associated with major congenital abnormalities (5.5%).[35] Lithium is a weak teratogen, associated with a small risk of cardiac abnormalities, as well as risk of toxicity in the neonate. The newer antiepileptic and mood stabilizers lamotrigine and levatirecetam are safer alternatives compared to the aforementioned medications.[31]

Women of reproductive age taking known teratogenic drugs or drugs with potential teratogenic effects must always be advised to use highly effective contraception (such as Cu-IUD, levonorg-estrel intrauterine system or progestogen-only implant).

Detailed information regarding teratogenic drugs is available from the UK Teratology Information Service (UKTIS) website (www.uktis.org).[37]

Metabolic side effects

Second-generation antipsychotics are associated with metabolic side effects, including hypertension, dyslipidaemia, diabetes, obesity, embolism and thrombosis.[38] It is worth noting that regardless of antipsychotic treatment, individuals with mental illness are significantly more likely to develop and die prematurely from cardiovascular disease.[39,40] Rates of obesity are greater in patients with bipolar affective disorder compared to controls.[41] There are also higher rates of smoking in individuals with mental illness. Several of these are contraindications for hormonal contraceptives. Effectiveness of the emergency contraceptive levonorgestrel could be reduced in individuals with weight over 70 kg/BMI greater than 26 kg/m^2.[42] It is also important to note the DMPA contraceptive injection is associated with weight gain. Metabolic side effects are thus important considerations for clinicians when choosing appropriate contraception for patients with mental illness.

Osteoporosis

Antipsychotics and opiates can cause hyperprolactinaemia which in turn may lead to osteoporosis and fractures.[43] In individuals taking these medications, the DMPA injection may not be a good option due to the associated increased risk of osteoporosis.

Oligo/amenorrhoea

Women on antipsychotic drugs, heroin or methadone are often amenorrhoeic. Amenorrhoea may also result from eating disorders, such as anorexia nervosa. The evaluation of this is no different from that of other women. Patients may not use contraception because they mistakenly think they are infertile when their periods become absent or irregular. It is important to counsel women in their reproductive years that they have not experienced premature menopause and are still capable of becoming pregnant.[6]

Use of sodium valproate has been associated with polycystic ovary syndrome (PCOS). Women with PCOS are higher risk of developing endometrial cancer and should be recommended an IUS for endometrial protection.[44] Contraceptive implants have not been shown to provide effective endometrial protection in women with PCOS and oral contraception is not effective enough given the teratogenicity of sodium valproate. Contraceptive injections protect the endometrium and are effective if given regularly but can cause weight gain.

Effect of hormonal contraception on mental health

There is conflicting evidence regarding the association of hormonal contraception with depression.

Two large retrospective cohort studies in Denmark of women with no past use of contraceptive hormones and no current or past MH problems showed that contraceptive hormones increase the risk of a depression diagnosis, starting antidepressive medication[45] and attempted and completed suicide.[46] Taking the two studies from Denmark together, there was no clinically relevant difference between different contraceptive hormones, different doses and routes of administration. Systematic reviews did not show that hormonal contraception affects the incidence[47,48] or course[49] of depression. The general consensus is that it is not proven that contraceptive hormones cause depression.[50] Nonetheless, an effect on mood of contraceptive hormones is biologically plausible[51] and cannot be ignored. If a woman reports that her mood has deteriorated after starting hormonal contraception, she should be offered an IUD or switch to a different hormonal contraceptive or route of administration. Injectable contraception cannot be removed, and as it may take up to a year to clear from the body, it would be better to avoid in women who are already reporting mood problems with contraceptive hormones in the past.

Depression is the only MH problem addressed by WHO MEC (the World Health Organization medical eligibility criteria),[52] UK-MEC[53] and USMEC.[54] It is a category 1 condition for all reversible methods of contraception (no restriction for use).

Ethical and legal considerations

Mental capacity and consent

Most people with SMI have the same ability as people without SMI to make contraceptive decisions. A woman's decision to discontinue a LARC method may be unwise, but we nonetheless need to assume that she is competent to request this and her autonomous decision not to take emergency contraception or to start or to discontinue contraception should be respected. Contraceptive coercion or deception must always be avoided. Anything else would not respect her sexual and reproductive health care rights.

Women with SMI will be aware that sometimes they are making an unreasonable decision and may wish to safeguard against this by making a Ulysses contract.[55] This is legal agreement to override a present request from a legally competent patient in favour of a past request made by that patient, for example, to have emergency contraception on admission with a manic illness, provided the pregnancy test is negative or not to remove a LARC if requesting this during a psychotic episode.[19] Where competence is in doubt, permission should be obtained to discuss her situation with her MH team.

Safeguarding

Patients with mental illness are more vulnerable to sexual exploitation. Always enquire about sexual coercion, domestic violence and substance misuse in women of reproductive age, and raise safeguarding concerns when required.

Contraception, pregnancy planning and human rights

People with MH problems have the right to contraception and the right to a family. Women with chronic MH problems should be assisted to plan pregnancies when stable and have support for the pregnancy and puerperal period.

The role of SRH care is not merely to provide contraception but to enable women to realise their sexual and reproductive health rights. If we do not take this approach, patients may view us with suspicion, and we will not see those who will benefit most from our care. Barriers that reduce access to our services need to be addressed as a priority.

KEY POINTS

- Poor sexual and reproductive health (SRH) care has serious consequences for people with mental illness and for society

- Women of reproductive age should be routinely assessed for psychologic well-being, and screened for substance misuse and domestic violence

- Barriers to SRH services should be reduced for easier access

- Mental health patients should be assumed to be competent and their contraceptive decisions non-coercive and autonomous

- Enquire about pregnancy plans in women of reproductive age with mental illness, and discuss risk of unplanned pregnancy and contraception

- Long-acting reversible contraception should be advocated as they are highly effective nonuser-dependent methods

- Beware of drug interactions between certain contraceptives and psychotropic medications

- Ensure women of reproductive age who are taking teratogenic drugs have a pregnancy prevention plan in place

- Currently, there is conflicting evidence linking hormonal contraceptives with negative impact on mood

- Help individuals to optimise their chances of healthy pregnancy by providing preconception counselling

References

1. American Psychiatric Association. Diagnostic and Statistical Manual of Mental Disorders. Fifth Edition (DSM-5). Arlington, VA: American Psychiatric Association; 2013.
2. Robakis T, Williams KE, Nutkiewicz L, Rasgon NL. Hormonal contraceptives and mood: review of the literature and implications for future research. Curr Psychiatry Rep 2019;21(7):57.
3. Joffe H. Reproductive biology and psychotropic treatments in premenopausal women with bipolar disorder. J Clin Psychiatry 2007;68(Suppl.9):10–15.
4. Miller DE, Sebastian CS. Olanzapine-induced hyperprolactinemia and galactorrhea reversed with addition of bromocriptine: a case report. J Clin Psychiatry 2005;66(2):269–270.
5. Lusskin SI, Cancro R, Chuang L, Jacobson J. Prolactin elevation with ziprasidone. Am J Psychiatry 2004;161(10):1925.
6. Seeman MV, Ross R. Prescribing contraceptives for women with schizophrenia. J Psychiatr Pract 2011;17(4):258–269.
7. Marengo E, Martino DJ, Igoa A, Scápola M, Fassi G, Baamonde MU, et al. Unplanned pregnancies and reproductive health among women with bipolar disorder. J Affect Disord 2015;178:201–205.
8. Hubacher D, Spector H, Monteith C, Chen PL, Hart C. Long-acting reversible contraceptive acceptability and unintended pregnancy among women presenting for short-acting methods: a randomized patient preference trial. Am J Obstet Gynecol 2017;216(2):101–109.
9. Rasgon NL, Kenna HA, Reynolds-May MF, Stemmle PG, Vemuri M, Marsh W, et al. Metabolic dysfunction in women with bipolar disorder: the potential influence of family history of type 2 diabetes mellitus. Bipolar Disord 2010;12(5):504–513.

10. Burt VK, Bernstein C, Rosenstein WS, Altshuler LL. Bipolar disorder and pregnancy: maintaining psychiatric stability in the real world of obstetric and psychiatric complications. Am J Psychiatry 2010;167(8):892–897.

11. Newport DJ, Stowe ZN, Viguera AC, Calamaras MR, Juric S, Knight B, et al. Lamotrigine in bipolar disorder: efficacy during pregnancy. Bipolar Disord 2008;10(3):432–436.

12. NatCen Social Research and the Department of Health Sciences, University of Leicester. Mental Health and Wellbeing in England Adult Psychiatric Morbidity Survey 2014. NHS Digital 2014. https://files.digital.nhs.uk/pdf/q/3/mental_health_and_wellbeing_in_england_full_report.pdf.

13. Callegari LS, Zhao X, Nelson KM, Borrero S. Contraceptive adherence among women Veterans with mental illness and substance use disorder. Contraception 2015;91(5):386–392.

14. Canfield M, Radcliffe P, Marlow S, Boreham M, Gilchrist G. Maternal substance use and child protection: a rapid evidence assessment of factors associated with loss of child care. Child Abuse Negl 2017;70:11–27.

15. Zacher L, Peterson J, Lempicki K, Zaror P. Comparing current practices of screening for pregnancy and contraceptive use in female veterans of child-bearing age prescribed psychotropic medications in a mental health versus a women's health clinic. Ment Health Clin 2013;3(2):71–77.

16. Coverdale JH, Aruffo JF. AIDS and family planning counseling of psychiatrically ill women in community mental health clinics. Community Ment Health J 1992; 28(1):13–20.

17. Coverdale J, Aruffo J, Grunebaum H. Developing family planning services for female chronic mentally ill outpatients. Hosp Community Psychiatry 1992;43(5):475–478.

18. National Institute for Health and Care Excellence (NICE). Recommendations | Antenatal and postnatal mental health: clinical management and service guidance | Guidance | NICE. (2014; updated in 2020). https://www.nice.org.uk/guidance/cg192/chapter/Key-priorities-for-implementation.

19. Kumar U, Pathak N. Maudsley guidelines: contraception and mental health. In: Taylor D, Gaughran F, Pillinger T, editors. The maudsley: practice guidelines for physical health conditions in psychiatry. London: Wiley Blackwell; 2020. pp. 307–316.

20. Miller LJ. Sexuality, reproduction, and family planning in women with schizophrenia. Schizophr Bull 1997;23(4):623–635.

21. Coverdale JH, Bayer TL, McCullough LB, Chervenak FA. Respecting the autonomy of chronic mentally ill women in decisions about contraception. Hosp Community Psychiatry 1993;44(7):671–674.

22. Stodieck SRG, Schwenkhagen AM. Lamotrigine plasma levels and combined monophasic oral contraceptives or a contraceptive vaginal ring, a prospective evaluation in 30 women. Epilepsia 2004;45(Suppl. 7):187.

23. Schwenkhagen AM, Stodieck SRG. Interaction between lamotrigine and progesten-only contraceptive pill containing desogestrel 75 μg (Cerazette). Epilepsia 2004;45(Suppl. 7):154.

24. Gabbay V, O'Dowd MA, Mamamtavrishvili M, Asnis GM. Clozapine and oral contraceptives: a possible drug interaction. J Clin Psychopharmacol 2002;22(6):621–622.

25. Brown D, Goosen TC, Chetty M, Hamman JH. Effect of oral contraceptives on the transport of chlorpromazine across the CACO-2 intestinal epithelial cell line. Eur J Pharm Biopharm 2003;56(2):159–165.

26. Chetty M, Miller R. Oral contraceptives increase the plasma concentrations of chlorpromazine. Ther Drug Monit 2001;23(5):556–568.

27. The Faculty of Sexual and Reproductive Healthcare (FSRH). Clinical Effectiveness Unit (CEU) Clinical Guidance: Drug Interactions with Hormonal Contraception. (2017, last reviewed 2019). https://www.fsrh.org/documents/ceu-clinical-guidance-drug-interactions-with-hormonal/.

28. British National Formulary (BNF). www.bnf.org.

29. Medicines Complete. Stockley's Drug Interactions. www.medicinescomplete.com/mc/index.htm.

30. Electronic Medicine Compendium. www.medicines.org.uk/emc.
31. Ornoy A, Weinstein-Fudim L, Ergaz Z. Antidepressants, antipsychotics, and mood stabilizers in pregnancy: what do we know and how should we treat pregnant women with depression. Birth Defects Res 2017;109(12):933–956.
32. Ban L, Gibson JE, West J, Fiaschi L, Sokal R, Smeeth L, et al. Maternal depression, antidepressant prescriptions, and congenital anomaly risk in offspring: a population-based cohort study. BJOG 2014;121(12):1471–1481.
33. Huybrechts KF, Hernández-Díaz S, Patorno E, Desai RJ, Mogun H, Dejene SZ, et al. Antipsychotic use in pregnancy and the risk for congenital malformations. JAMA Psychiatry 2016;73(9):938–946.
34. Grigoriadis S, VonderPorten EH, Mamisashvili L, Roerecke M, Rehm J, Dennis CL, et al. Antidepressant exposure during pregnancy and congenital malformations: is there an association? A systematic review and meta-analysis of the best evidence. J Clin Psychiatry 2013;74(4):e293–e308.
35. Vossler DG. Comparative risk of major congenital malformations with 8 different antiepileptic drugs: a prospective cohort study of the EURAP Registry. Epilepsy Curr 2019;19(2):83–85.
36. Medicines and Healthcare products Regulatory Agency. MHRA Drug Safety Update 2020;13(7):1–16. https://assets.publishing.service.gov.uk/government/uploads/system/uploads/attachment_data/file/865491/Feb-2020-PDF.pdf.
37. UK Teratology Information Service (UKTIS). www.uktis.org.
38. Hirsch L, Patten SB, Bresee L, Jette N, Pringsheim T. Second-generation antipsychotics and metabolic side-effects: Canadian population-based study. BJPsych Open 2018;4(4):256–261.
39. Harris EC, Barraclough B. Excess mortality of mental disorder. Br J Psychiatry 1998;173(1):11–53.
40. Laursen TM, Munk-Olsen T, Vestergaard M. Life expectancy and cardiovascular mortality in persons with schizophrenia. Curr Opin Psychiatry 2012;25(2):83–88.
41. Goldstein BI, Liu SM, Zivkovic N, Schaffer A, Chien LC, Blanco C. The burden of obesity among adults with bipolar disorder in the United States. Bipolar Disord 2011;13(4):387–395.
42. The Faculty of Sexual & Reproductive Healthcare of the Royal College of Obstetricians & Gynaecologists (FSRH). FSRH Guideline Emergency Contraception. 2017. https://www.fsrh.org/standards-and-guidance/documents/ceu-clinical-guidance-emergency-contraception-march-2017/.
43. De Hert M, Detraux J, Stubbs B. Relationship between antipsychotic medication, serum prolactin levels and osteoporosis/osteoporotic fractures in patients with schizophrenia: a critical literature review. Expert Opin Drug Saf 2016;15(6):809–823.
44. Bilo L, Meo R. Polycystic ovary syndrome in women using valproate: a review. Gynecol Endocrinol 2008;24(10):562–570.
45. Skovlund CW, Mørch LS, Kessing LV, Lidegaard Ø. Association of hormonal contraception with depression. JAMA Psychiatry 2016;73(11):1154-62.
46. Skovlund CW, Mørch LS, Kessing LV, Lange T, Lidegaard Ø. Association of hormonal contraception with suicide attempts and suicides. Am J Psychiatry 2018;175(4):336–342.
47. Worly BL, Gur TL, Schaffir J. The relationship between progestin hormonal contraception and depression: a systematic review. Contraception 2018;97(6):478–489.
48. Schaffir J, Worly BL, Gur TL. Combined hormonal contraception and its effects on mood: a critical review. Eur J Contracept Reprod Health Care 2016;21(5):347–355.
49. Pagano HP, Zapata LB, Berry-Bibee EN, Nanda K, Curtis KM. Safety of hormonal contraception and intrauterine devices among women with depressive and bipolar disorders: a systematic review. Contraception 2016;94(6):641–649.
50. The Faculty of Sexual & Reproductive Healthcare (FSRH) Clinical Effectiveness Unit. CEU response to published study: Association of Hormonal Contraception with Depression. October 4, 2016. https://www.fsrh.org/documents/ceu-response-to-published-study-association-of-hormonal/.

51. Gingnell M, Engman J, Frick A, Moby L, Wikström J, Fredrikson M, et al. Oral contraceptive use changes brain activity and mood in women with previous negative affect on the pill—a double-blinded, placebo-controlled randomized trial of a levonorgestrel-containing combined oral contraceptive. Psychoneuroendocrinology 2013;38(7):1133–1144.
52. World Health Organization (WHO). Medical eligibility criteria for contraceptive use. 5th edition. 2015. https://www.who.int/reproductivehealth/publications/family_planning/Ex-Summ-MEC-5/en/.
53. The Faculty of Sexual & Reproductive Healthcare of the Royal College of Obstetricians & Gynaecologists (FSRH). FSRH UK Medical Eligibility Criteria for Contraceptive Use; UKMEC 2016 (AMENDED SEPTEMBER 2019). 2019. https://www.fsrh.org/ukmec/.
54. Centers for Disease Control and Prevention. US Medical Eligibility Criteria (US MEC) for Contraceptive Use, 2016. 2016. https://www.cdc.gov/reproductivehealth/contraception/mmwr/mec/summary.html.
55. Standing H, Lawlor R. Ulysses Contracts in psychiatric care: helping patients to protect themselves from spiralling. J Med Ethics 2019;45(11):693–699.

APPENDIX A

The UK Medical Eligibility Criteria for Contraceptive Use

UK medical eligibility criteria (UKMEC) 2016 (amended September 2019), adapted from the World Health Organization (WHO) guidelines (WHO Medical Eligibility Criteria for Contraceptive Use, WHOMEC 5th edition) offer guidance to healthcare professionals regarding safe use of contraception.[1] It provides information about possible methods that can be used safely for contraceptive purposes by individuals with certain health conditions or characteristics. UKMEC categories do not reflect the efficacy of methods which may be affected by the condition or a medication required for the condition. The UKMEC considers the following group of contraceptive methods: intrauterine contraception (IUC), progestogen only contraception (POC), combined hormonal contraception (CHC) and emergency contraception (EC).

For each of the personal characteristics or medical conditions, a category 1, 2, 3 or 4 is given.[1] The definitions of these categories are given in Table Appendix 1.1.

Table Appendix 1.1

Definition of UK medical eligibility criteria categories	
UK medical eligibility criteria	**Definition of category**
Category 1	A condition for which there is no restriction for the use of the method
Category 2	A condition where the advantages of using the method generally outweigh the theoretical or proven risks
	Continued

Table Appendix 1.1

Definition of UK medical eligibility criteria categories—cont'd

UK medical eligibility criteria	Definition of category
Category 3	A condition where the theoretical or proven risks usually outweigh the advantages of using the method. The provision of a method requires expert clinical judgement and/or referral to a specialist contraceptive provider, since use of the method is not usually recommended unless other, more appropriate methods are not available or not acceptable
Category 4	A condition which represents an unacceptable health risk if the method is used

1. Faculty of Sexual and Reproductive Healthcare 2016 (Amended September 2019) *UK Medical Eligibility Criteria for Contraceptive Use.* [The full version of the UKMEC 2016 guidance can be accessed from https://www.fsrh.org/ukmec/]
Reproduced under licence from FSRH. Copyright ©Faculty of Sexual and Reproductive Healthcare December 2017.

APPENDIX B

Contraception Choices and Effectiveness of Contraceptive Methods

A wide range of contraceptive methods are available with varying effectiveness. Table Appendix 2.1 compares the percentage of women experiencing an unintended pregnancy during the first year of contraceptive use when the method is used 'typically' (which includes both incorrect and inconsistent use) or 'perfectly' (correct and consistent use).[1] Effectiveness varies widely between 'typical' and 'perfect' use for the methods that require consistent and correct use by the user. User-independent methods such as the long-acting reversible contraceptives (LARC) (copper intrauterine device [Cu-IUD], levonorgestrel intrauterine system [LNG-IUS] and the progestogen-only implant), female sterilisation and vasectomy are considered highly effective contraception, with a failure rate of less than 1% with 'typical' use. Progestogen-only injections may be considered as highly effective if repeat injections are administered on schedule. User-dependent methods such as the condom, diaphragm, fertility awareness-based methods, oral contraceptive pills, transdermal patch and vaginal ring are not considered highly effective because 'typical' use is associated with risk of failure.

Table Appendix 2.1

Percentage of women experiencing an unintended pregnancy during the first year of typical use and first year of perfect use of contraception		
Method	**Typical use (%)**	**Perfect use (%)**
No method	85	85
Withdrawal	20	4
Fertility awareness-based methods	15	0.4–5
Diaphragm	17	16

Table Appendix 2.1

Percentage of women experiencing an unintended pregnancy during the first year of typical use and first year of perfect use of contraception—cont'd

Method	Typical use (%)	Perfect use (%)
Male condom	13	2
Female condom	21	5
Combined hormonal contraception (CHC) (includes combined oral contraception, transdermal patch and vaginal ring)	7	0.3
Progestogen-only pill	7	0.3
Progestogen-only injectable (depo-medroxyproges-terone acetate [DMPA])	4	0.2
Copper-bearing intrauterine device (Cu-IUD)	0.8	0.6
Levonorgestrel-releasing intrauterine system (LNG-IUS)		
Mirena, Levosert (52 mg LNG)	0.1	0.1
Kyleena (19.5 mg LNG)	0.2	0.2
Jaydess (13.5 mg LNG)	0.4	0.3
Progestogen-only implant (Nexplanon)	0.1	0.1
Female sterilisation	0.5	0.5
Vasectomy	0.15	0.1

(Modified and reproduced with permission from: Trussell J, Aiken ARA. Contraceptive efficacy. In: Hatcher RA, Nelson AL, Trussell J, Cwiak C, Cason P, Policar MS, Edelman A, Aiken ARA, Marrazzo J, Kowal D, eds. Contraceptive technology. 21st ed. New York, NY: Ayer Company Publishers, Inc., 2018.)
Reproduced under licence from FSRH. Copyright © Faculty of Sexual and Reproductive Heathcare December 2017.

References

1. Trussel J, Aiken ARA. Contraceptive efficacy. In: Hatcher RA, Nelson AL, Trussell J, Cwiak C, Cason P, Policar MS, Edelman A, Aiken ARA, Marrazzo J, Kowal D, eds. *Contraceptive technology.* 21st ed. New York, NY: Ayer Company Publishers, Inc., 2018.

Index

Page numbers followed by "f" indicate figures, "t" indicate tables, and "b" indicate boxes.